MOBILITY

Patient Problems
and
Nursing Care

MOBILITY

Patient Problems and Nursing Care

Maggie Judd

RGN, ONC, RCNT, RNT, Cert Ed (F.E.)
*Tutor to ENB Courses 219 and 222
Avon School of Nursing
Bristol*

Illustrations by Jane Upton

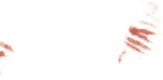

Heinemann Nursing

Heinemann Nursing
An imprint of Heinemann Professional Publishing Ltd
Halley Court, Jordan Hill, Oxford OX2 8EJ

OXFORD   LONDON   SINGAPORE   NAIROBI   IBADAN
KINGSTON

First published 1989

© Maggie Judd 1989

British Library Cataloguing in Publication Data
Judd, Maggie
  Mobility: patient problems and nursing care.
  1. Immobilised patients. Nursing
  I. Title
  610.73
  ISBN 0–433–001674

Photoset by Wilmaset, Birkenhead, Wirral
Printed in Great Britain by
Biddles Ltd, Guildford and Kings Lynn

Contents

Preface vii

Chapter 1 Mobility 1
Chapter 2 Immobility 9
Chapter 3 Nursing care and the assessment of immobility 30
Chapter 4 The patient suffering temporary immobilization 45
Chapter 5 The patient with permanent immobility of gradual onset 74
Chapter 6 The patient with permanent immobility of sudden onset 109
Chapter 7 Care of the child with a mobility problem 133
Chapter 8 The immobile individual in the community 163

Index 185

Dedication

To Bethan, Ben and Mike, with all my love.

Preface

Some people say that there is a book within us all waiting to be written. I didn't believe that before I started this book and I certainly don't believe it now.

However the fact that it has been written is due to the many people who have influenced and helped me throughout my nursing career, from my days as a prebasic student in the Bath & Wessex Orthopaedic Hospital, through my general training at the Bristol Royal Infirmary, my experiences as a ward sister in the trauma unit at the BRI and as a teacher in the Avon School of Nursing. My thanks go to you all.

On a personal note I would like to thank my mother who provided a wonderful role model and showed me how worthwhile caring for others can be. I would also like to thank my brothers Peter, David and Anthony and their families for their love and support whenever I needed it and my children Bethan and Ben who have managed to bring me up as a mother very well – against all the odds!

Susan Devlin and the staff of Heinemanns deserve my thanks and praise for tackling my references and bringing them into order. I would also like to thank Ann Lawrence, Learning Resources Manager, Avon School of Nursing for her help in researching the literature and generally listening to me when it all seemed too much.

Finally, of course, I must thank Mike Walsh, the Series Editor in whom I have met my match for enthusiasm. It is only through his persuading, coercing and finally blatant nagging tactics that the manuscript was completed. He also bought the beer that night in 'The George' when the framework of this book was conceived. What more can I say!

Maggie Judd

1
Mobility

The *Oxford Illustrated Dictionary* defines mobility as that which is characterized by freedom of movement or that which can be easily moved from place to place.

To be able to move at will is regarded by most as an essential part of living. However, consider those aged over 65 years who live in the community. Of these, 43% require help in their daily lives mainly due to a problem of mobility (Levine, 1969). Add to this the number of postoperative surgical patients in hospital, those with a progressive neurological condition who require help with mobility and those who, due to trauma, have been transformed overnight from being active and healthy to requiring help in the most basic of movements, and it will be easy to see the size of the problem.

Whatever means is used to assess a patient with a mobility problem, it has to be appreciated that the terms 'ambulant' and 'mobile' are not synonymous. (In the *Collins Dictionary*, ambulant is defined as walking while mobile is defined as easily moved). A patient may be mobile in bed but only able to move outside it in a wheelchair. On the other hand, an individual who has had a total hip replacement may be immobilized in bed but able to walk around the ward.

When care is being planned and goals set, it is essential that the nurse uses the patient's perspective of the problem. Most nurses, because of the very nature of their work, are fit and may therefore be guilty of a lack of realism in their expectations of patient mobility.

The two basic anatomical units required for movement are

2 MOBILITY

nerves and muscles. Together with bones, which act as joints and levers, they are responsible for movements as different as the fingering of a concert violinist and the thrust of an olympic weightlifter. The weakest points of the musculoskeletal system are the joints, and it is the wear and tear on these which is responsible for many problems of mobility, especially in the elderly.

THE ANATOMY OF JOINTS

Although, traditionally, joints have been divided into three groups (fixed, slightly movable and freely movable), for the sake of brevity only the freely movable, synovial joint will be discussed here. Most of the joints involved in maintaining mobility fall into this category.

A joint occurs where two bones meet and, in this case move (see Fig. 1.1.). To facilitate movement, the surfaces of the

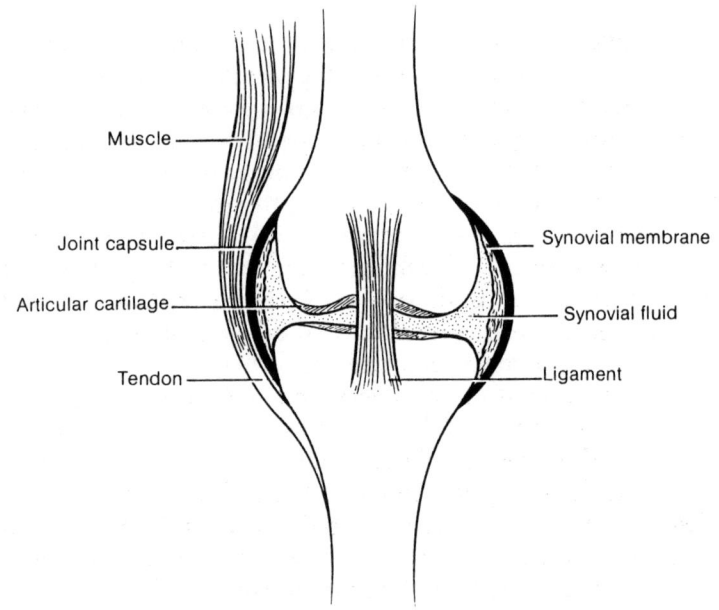

Fig. 1.1 *A typical synovial joint*

bones which come into contact are covered in smooth hyaline (articular) cartilage. This tissue lacks the rigidity of bone but has the strength to bear the full weight on the joint. It is the deterioration of the hyaline cartilage that results in osteoarthritis. Enclosing the whole joint is the joint capsule which is strengthened by ligaments and lined by the synovial membrane. The secretory epithelium which comprises the synovial membrane produces fluid similar in consistency to the white of an egg. This fluid is essential to protect the hyaline cartilage and act as a shock absorber in the joint, rather as oil does in a machine. Sacs of synovial fluid (bursae) are also found in some joints preventing friction between bone and tendons or ligaments. Rheumatoid arthritis is a systemic condition in which the synovial membrane is affected such that the joint becomes deformed, sometimes becoming fixed in an abnormal position.

NEUROMUSCULAR PHYSIOLOGY

For voluntary movement to occur, an impulse must travel from the cerebral cortex, down the pyramidal tracts to the anterior horn in the spinal cord (upper motor neuron). The lower motor neuron is the path along which the impulse travels from the anterior horn to the muscle fibre (see Fig. 1.2). All such movements are modified by the presence of a supplementary pathway originating in several areas of the brain below conscious level, including the basal ganglia and the cerebellum. A condition in which this extrapyramidal tract is affected results in abnormal movements such as the tremors seen in Parkinson's disease.

The point at which the nerve and muscle fibres meet is termed the neuromuscular junction (see Fig. 1.3). The end of the lower motor neuron flattens out to form the motor end-plate which lies in apposition with the end-plate receptors of the muscle fibre. When a nerve impulse reaches the motor end-plate, the chemical transmitter acetylcholine is released and becomes attached to the receptors in the muscle. Thus, the impulse crosses the gap and the muscle is able to contract. The action of acetylcholine is stopped by the enzyme cholin-

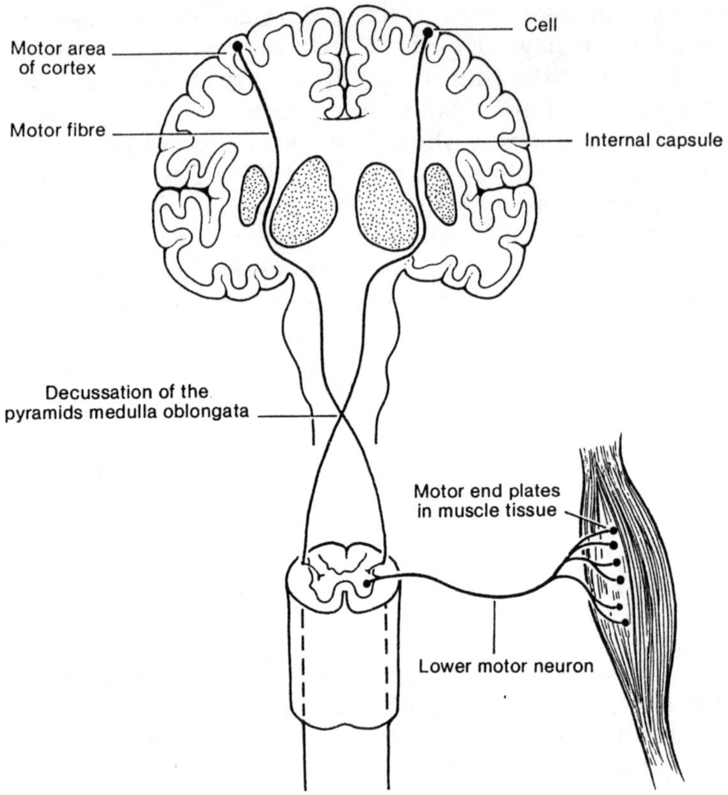

4 MOBILITY

Fig. 1.2 *The upper and lower motor neurons*

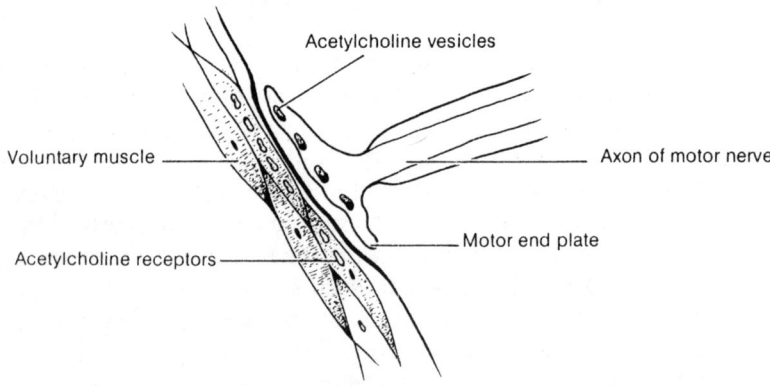

Fig. 1.3 *A neuromuscular junction*

esterase which is released from vesicles near the end-plate receptors.

Muscles responsible for voluntary movement are described as striped because of their microscopic appearance of alternate light and dark bands. These bands are composed of the proteins actin and myosin. The muscle fibre shortens and thickens in isotonic contraction, but will simply increase in tension in isometric contraction. The strength of the muscle contraction depends on the total number of muscle fibres involved, as each fibre works on an 'all or nothing' principle.

HOW MOVEMENT OCCURS

To allow the movement of limbs, both ends of a muscle need to be attached to different jointed bones by a tendon. As the muscle contracts and shortens, the two ends of the muscle are brought nearer together and hence one of the bones will move (see Fig. 1.4). The tendons which attach the muscles to the bones are referred to as the tendons of origin and insertion. Generally, the proximal tendon is the origin and the distal tendon the insertion. The muscles around a joint work in pairs; the one that contracts to bring about movement is termed the agonist whereas the muscle which relaxes in cooperation is termed the antagonist.

The long bones of the limbs act as levers allowing an arc of movement proportionate to their length. Consequently, a child with shorter legs has to run to keep up with the walking pace of an adult.

For walking to occur, the body weight needs to be transferred from one leg to the other. As the moving body passes over the supporting leg, the other leg must swing forward for the next support phase. One foot is always on the ground, and the body weight is systematically transferred from the trailing to the leading leg. There is a short time during which both feet are on the ground. When a patient is learning the rudiments of walking following a period of immobility, both feet may be on the ground for longer than usual to help maintain balance. However, as walking becomes faster, this period shortens until it is lost altogether, as in running when it is replaced by short periods with neither foot on the ground.

6 MOBILITY

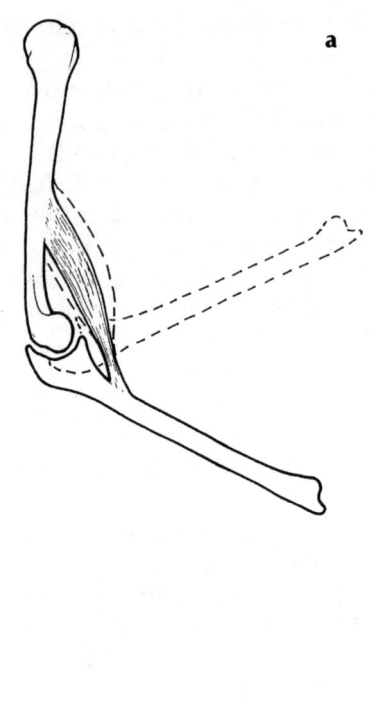

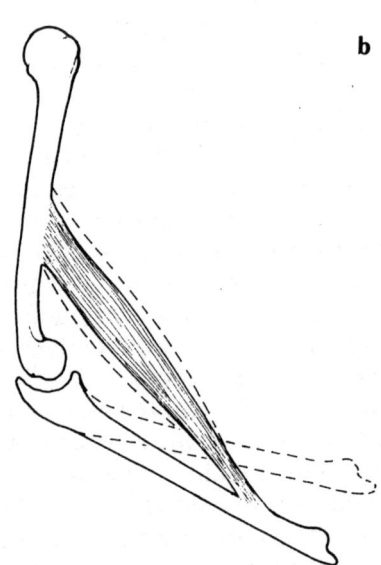

Fig. 1.4 *Diagrams to show how bones act as levers*

Walking is a learned activity; the congenitally blind child never spontaneously attempts to walk or stand but has to be taught. Similarly, many individuals have to learn to walk again using new techniques and acquiring new skills (for example, using a prosthesis following an amputation, or relying on two crutches rather than one leg during a period of non-weight bearing after a fracture of the lower limb).

'Gait' is a term used frequently by physiotherapists and nurses who are specifically concerned with teaching individuals to walk again. It is a more specific term than 'walking' and refers to the overall pattern of locomotion, the movement of other parts of the body which help in walking (for example, rotation of the body at the trunk and hips) and the economic use of energy. Gait can be analysed by:
1. Listening to the patient describe their problems with walking
2. Watching the patient walk
3. Breaking the gait down into a series of events, and considering the range of joint movement and the timing of each part of the sequence.

SUMMARY

We can see that mobility involves the correct functioning of both the central and peripheral nervous system together with the musculoskeletal system. Damage to either of these components, such as a cerebrovascular accident or disease of the joints, will therefore seriously impair mobility.

If we consider for a while the whole patient rather than just the mechanics of movement, we see that the term 'mobility' describes a highly complex state of being which is easily lost. When this occurs, the effect on the individual is much more than simply inability to move at will. Bernal, in her essay on *Immobility and the Self* (Bernal, 1984), investigates the notion that the 'lived body' is a means of perceiving the world and expressing one's individuality; lose it (as happens to the immobile) and part of this individuality is lost. Baird (1985) describes the negative connotations of being immobile that have been emphasized by society's demand for the ideals of youthfulness, wholeness and beauty. Those who are immobile are often unable to meet those ideals and consequently develop reduced opinions of themselves.

As the various aspects of nursing the patient with mobility problems are explored, the effects on the individual's self esteem and self perception will be dealt with in detail.

References

Baird S. (1985). Development of a nursing assessment tool to diagnose altered body image in immobilised patients. *Orthopaedic Nursing*, 4 (1), 47–53.

Bernal E. (1984). Immobility and the self; a clinical-existential inquiry. *Journal of Medicine and Philosophy*, 9, 75–91.

Levine M.E. (1969). The pursuit of wholeness. *American Journal of Nursing*, 69, 93–98.

Bibliography

Downie P. ed. (1984). *Cash's Textbook of Orthopaedics and Rheumatology for Physiotherapists*. London: Faber and Faber.

Green J.H. (1978). *An Introduction to Human Physiology* 4th edn. Oxford: Oxford University Press.

Watson J. (1979). *Medical-Surgical Nursing and Related Physiology*. Philadelphia: W.B. Saunders.

2
Immobility

The many pathological changes that cause immobility can be simplified into three broad categories:
1. Changes in some part of the nervous system resulting in the lack of muscle stimulation. This may be due to the inability of the cerebrum to initiate the impulse, a fault in the cerebellum which refines purposeful movement or a breakdown in the relay system linking the cerebrum with the muscles that help to bring about the movement.
2. Changes in muscle tissue leading to a state of permanent contraction (spasticity) or permanent relaxation (flaccidity).
3. Changes in the joints which may prevent any movement between the articular surfaces. This situation may be preceded by the individual voluntarily becoming immobile because of the pain caused by moving diseased joints.

The motor area of the brain which governs the initiation of voluntary movement lies just anterior to the central sulcus of the cerebrum (see Fig. 2.1). Both cerebral hemispheres have such a motor area, and it should be noted that the motor cortex (area) on each hemisphere controls the movement on the opposite side of the body. Damage to this part of the brain will result in the loss of voluntary movement either temporarily or permanently. Following a head injury or a cerebrovascular accident, there may be widespread loss of movement initially. This may recover, but the extent of recovery is highly variable, lying anywhere between a complete return of function and total lack of function.

10 MOBILITY

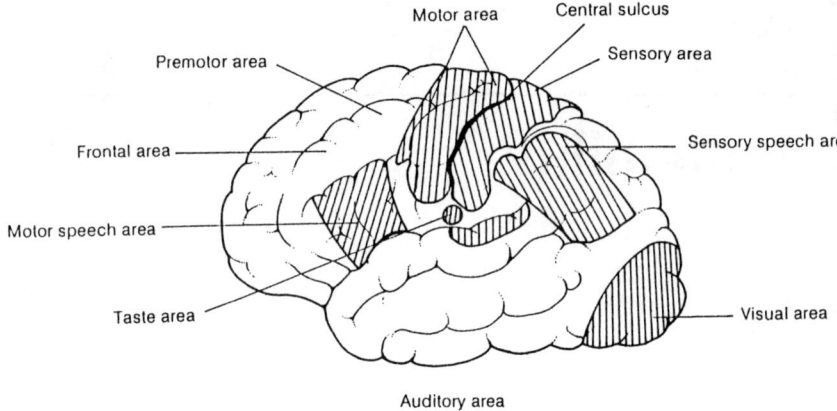

Fig. 2.1 *The functional areas of the cerebrum*

The control of movement of individual parts of the body lies in specific areas of the motor cortex known as the homunculus. The body is represented upside down with a large area devoted to the hands and face, ensuring the performance of intricate movements of the fingers and the mouth (see Fig. 2.2).

We have already mentioned that two of the most common ways in which damage to the motor area of the cerebrum can occur are following a cerebrovascular accident or head injury. The pathological changes behind these two situations will now be looked at in more detail, in addition to those which occur in a patient with a brain tumour.

CEREBROVASCULAR ACCIDENT

A cerebrovascular accident is a syndrome characterized as a sudden, non-convulsive onset of neurological deficits related directly or indirectly to a deficiency of the cerebral blood supply (Hickey, 1981). It is generally regarded as the third largest cause of death in Western civilization, following only heart disease and cancer. Neurological deficit may be manifest anywhere along a spectrum from slight tingling in a finger to complete loss of consciousness and death.

Cerebrovascular accident implies a deficiency in the cere-

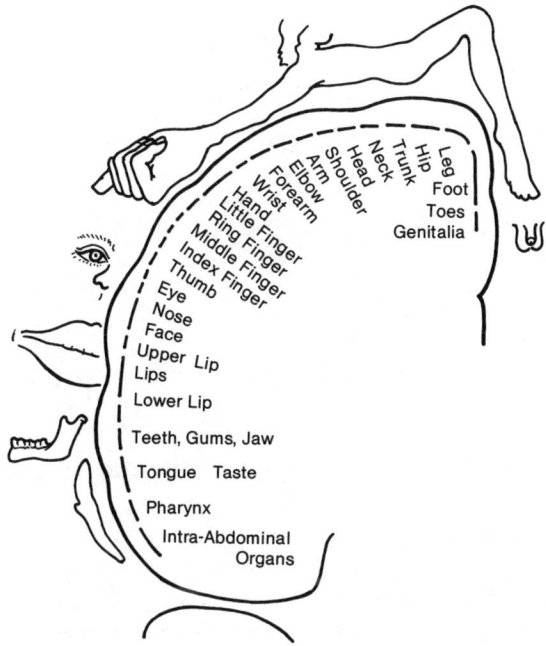

Fig. 2.2 *The motor homonculus*

bral blood supply. This may be due to a thrombus, haemorrhage or embolism in the vertebral, internal carotid, basilar or cerebral arteries or in the circle of Willis (see Fig. 2.3).

Cerebral thrombosis, like thrombosis in other parts of the body, is associated with atherosclerosis in which the lumen of the artery is narrowed, slowing the blood flow and leading to the formation of thrombi. Other conditions causing a slowing down of the arterial supply (statis), such as cardiac failure and shock, also predispose to the formation of thrombi. Once the vessel becomes occluded, the area of cerebral tissue it supplied becomes necrotic unless an alternative blood supply is available. Eventually, it will be replaced by scar tissue. The onset of a cerebral thrombosis is usually gradual, often when the victim is at rest.

Cerebral haemorrhage also may be associated with atherosclerosis which can cause degeneration of the arterial wall, and it commonly follows a long history of hypertension. The presence of an aneurysm (a weak saccular area in the vessel

12 MOBILITY

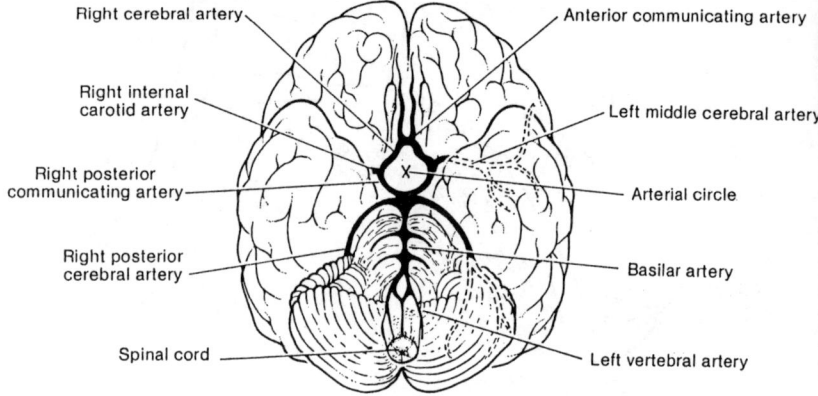

Fig. 2.3 *The blood supply to the brain from the circle of Willis*

wall) will also weaken the vessel wall and may lead to its rupture. A haematoma forms around the leaking blood vessel causing pressure on, and eventually death of, the surrounding brain tissue. This situation usually occurs suddenly when the victim is involved in some energetic pursuit or under great emotional strain.

An embolism is often a piece of thrombus which has broken free and is circulating on its own, but it may also be a piece of fat, a tiny particle of tumour or bacteria. A cerebral embolism is frequently the result of heart disease. A thrombus within the heart may break up and fragments enter the circulation. Thrombi from the internal carotid arteries are also common. Occasionally, cerebral embolism may be due to a fat embolism following a fracture of the femur or pelvis. An embolism due to bacteria would follow bacterial endocarditis. A cerebrovascular accident caused by an embolism is frequently of sudden onset.

As oxygen and glucose are the two essential requirements for cerebral metabolism, a continual blood supply is essential. Following a cerebrovascular accident, an area of the brain is deprived of its blood supply, resulting in necrosis. When this affects a part of the motor area, there will be loss of voluntary movement on the opposite side of the body.

HEAD INJURY

This term covers a variety of conditions including a fractured skull, brain injuries (concussion, contusion and lacerations of cranial tissue) and intercranial haemorrhage.

The overall effect of a brain injury will depend on which part of the brain is injured and the severity of the damage.

Cerebral oedema is a major problem following brain injuries as it can lead to infarction of further brain tissue. It results from a reduction in the tone of local arterioles which allows them to dilate and carry more blood. The result is increased pressure in the capillaries and venules, producing more movement of fluid into the tissues. This situation is exacerbated by inadequate sodium pump activity which leads to an accumulation of sodium and water in the brain cells. Raised cerebral carbon dioxide levels further contribute to cerebral oedema.

As cerebral oedema increases, the effect is to raise intracranial pressure which in turn leads to tentorial herniation. This phenomenon is the downward displacement of the cerebral hemispheres through the tentorial notch, compressing the mid-brain and brain stem (see Fig. 2.4) and eventually resulting in death.

For more information about the immediate care of patients who have undergone major head injuries, the reader is directed to a source particularly concerned with that topic.

Haemorrhage following head injuries may be extradural, subdural or intracerebral. Haematoma formation will cause an increase in intracranial pressure and may again result in infarction of areas of the brain. The effect of a haematoma is much the same as any space-occupying lesion. As the mass of brain tissue is displaced by the forming haematoma, cranial nerves and blood vessels may be bruised or torn. The most commonly affected cranial nerves are the oculomotor and optic nerves (see Fig. 2.5). Intracranial pressure will rise as the haematoma expands, and many eventually lead to tentorial herniation if nothing is done surgically (e.g. burr holes) to relieve the pressure.

Chronic subdural haematomas may develop very slowly following comparatively minor head injuries and may not be diagnosed until the patient becomes drowsy or develops a

14 MOBILITY

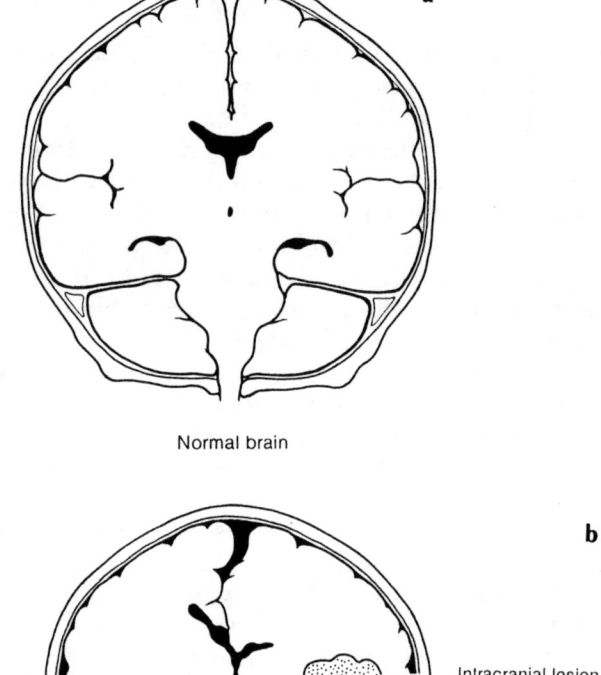

Fig. 2.4 *Tentorial herniation of the temporal lobe and brain stem due to intracranial lesion*

hemiparesis. In the elderly, such symptoms may be even slower to develop as these patients, due to cerebral atrophy, have more free space in their skulls which needs to be filled before the signs of raised intracranial pressure appear.

To prevent the serious complications of raised intracranial pressure, a haematoma will need to be evacuated through burr holes (small drill holes made in the skull) if possible. Sometimes, a craniotomy is indicated because the length of time

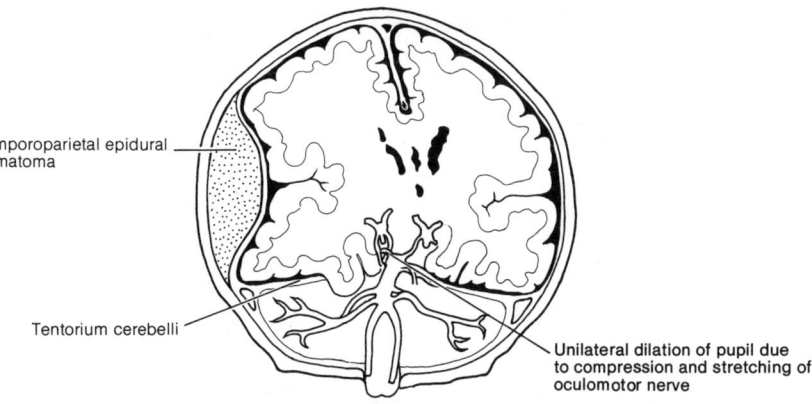

Fig. 2.5 *Cerebral haematoma causing unequal pupil reaction*

since injury has caused the clot to become too gelatinous to remove via burr holes.

BRAIN TUMOURS

Brain tumours account for approximately 2% of all cancer deaths (Hickey, 1981), but are responsible for much disability that is not evident from this figure. Secondary metastases from tumours elsewhere are the most common form.

Tumours affect the brain either by compression or by infiltration of surrounding tissue. Whichever type of tumour exists, there will be a resulting increase in pressure, cerebral oedema and focal neurological deficits; for example, if there is direct pressure or infiltration of the motor area, the patient will demonstrate problems with voluntary movement.

The treatment of brain tumours may be one or any combination of radiotherapy, chemotherapy or surgery. Unfortunately, it is a fact that either to reach the tumour or to remove it in its entirety often necessitates the removal of comparatively large amounts of brain tissue. The patient may therefore be left with a large neurological deficit.

NEUROLOGICAL DISORDERS

To link the brain with the muscles, the body employs a relay system composed of neurons. In the motor system, most of these neurons are insulated with a myelin sheath (see Fig. 2.6)

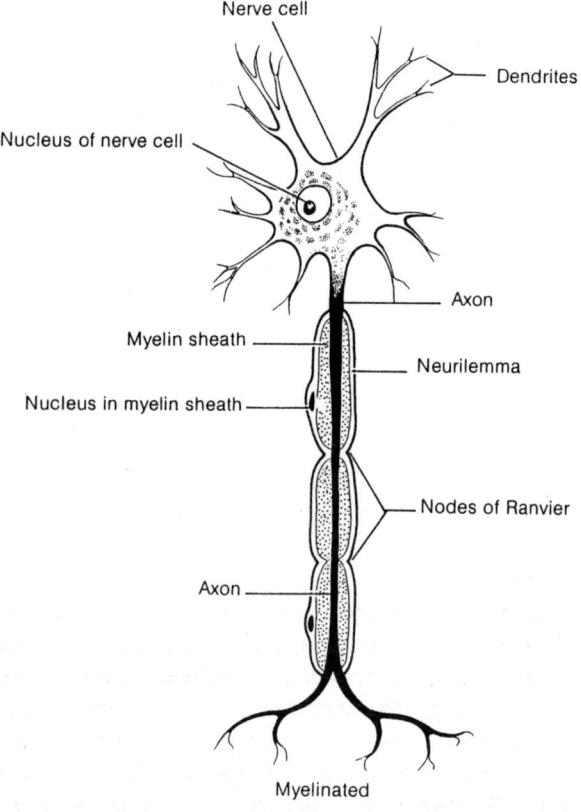

Fig. 2.6 *A myelinated nerve fibre*

which facilitates the speedy conduction of impulses. The transmission of a nerve impulse is highly complex, involving the exchange of sodium and potassium ions across the cell membrane and an alteration in the electrical state of the axon. This change from a negative to a positive state is known as an action potential.

In medullated nerve fibres (i.e. those with a myelin sheath) the action potential occurs at gaps in the sheath, called nodes of Ranvier. Thus, the impulse is able to 'leap' along the nerve fibre from node to node. For voluntary movement to occur, two neurons, conveniently termed the upper motor neuron and the lower motor neuron, are involved with the connection (synapse) in the spinal cord (see Fig. 2.7).

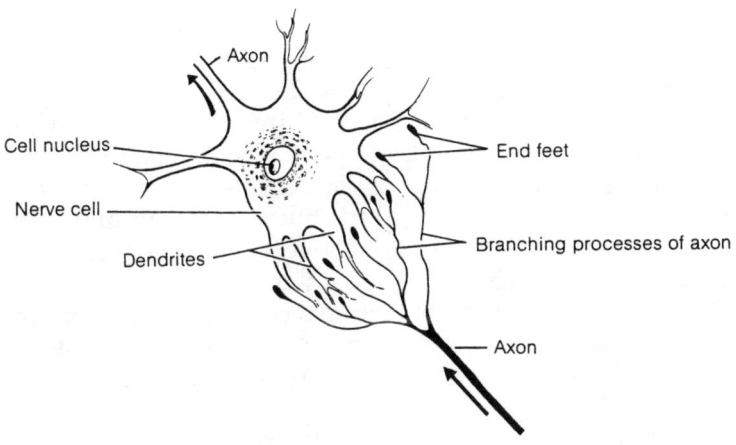

Fig. 2.7 A synapse

Situations which may interrupt this pathway include spinal cord injury following trauma, multiple sclerosis and poliomyelitis, a viral condition which destroys the myelin sheath leading to a flaccid paralysis. Multiple sclerosis affects the myelin sheath of the neuron by the deposition of sclerotic tissue along the axon, causing the death of the myelin. Eventually, the axon under the sclerosis dies and the patient is permanently paralysed. Before that stage is reached, the disease may be characterized by periods of remission when symptoms may disappear completely, but there is usually an overall downward trend. Once the neuron dies, and depending on its site, the patient may be left with a spastic paralysis of the limbs or a loss of sphincter control, or both.

Myasthenia gravis is a condition which affects the conduction of nerve impulses across the neuromuscular junction. It has been found that myasthenic patients have reduced quantities of acetylcholine and also a reduced number of acetylcholine receptor sites in the post synaptic membrane. These factors prevent muscle from contracting fully until eventually those muscle fibres which are contracting become exhausted and the muscle cannot contract at all.

There is some indication that myasthenia gravis falls under the 'umbrella' of auto-immune diseases (Macleod, 1981). This evidence is mainly circumstantial due to the association of myasthenia gravis with other auto-immune diseases such as rheumatoid arthritis and pernicious anaemia.

Specific pathological conditions of the muscular system are few, the one that is probably most familiar being muscular dystrophy. This condition is characterized by the symmetrical wasting of groups of muscles with no sensory loss.

There are three main types of muscular dystrophy. Each is inherited, although only the Duchenne type is transmitted by an X-linked recessive gene and therefore is almost exclusively found in males. The Erb type of muscular dystrophy is inherited as an autosomnal recessive gene; it usually appears in the second or third decade of life. Although the rate of progress of these two types of the disease is variable, death is likely before the age of forty.

The third type of muscular dystrophy is referred to as Landouzy-Déjérine and is a milder form. The periods of remission may be frequent and prolonged, and deterioration very slow.

There is no known cure for muscular dystrophy and treatment is aimed at keeping the patient as mobile as possible for as long as possible. Muscle contractures are a frequent occurrence and are kept at bay for as long as possible with the use of splints.

JOINTS

Pathological changes in joints are very common and account for the loss of mobility in a large proportion of the population. One in four patients who visit their general practitioner do so with an 'arthritic' problem (Wright and Haslock, 1984).

The two most common disorders of joints are osteoarthritis and rheumatoid arthritis. In the normal joint, the movement which occurs is aided by articular cartilage and synovial fluid.

Both these features are essential to the health of the joint, and when one or both become diseased, movements between the two bones become painful and consequently limited.

Osteoarthritis

In this disorder, the changes which occur in the articular (hyaline) cartilage have been traditionally attributed to old age and 'wear and tear'. However, although these two factors undoubtedly play a part, it is too simplistic to assume that only the elderly and obese are subject to osteoarthritis. Although weight-bearing joints such as hips and knees are highly susceptible to osteoarthritis and would support the 'load' theory, low load-bearing joints such as the distal interphalangeal joints are also commonly affected.

In the early stages of osteoarthritis, the surface of the articular cartilage becomes cracked and split, and the synovial membrane becomes inflamed. The cartilage is gradually lost, and osteophytes (small outgrowths of bone) are formed at the joint edges. The subchondral bone then becomes cystic in appearance due to the tracking of synovial fluid down the fissures in the cartilage (see Fig. 2.8). These three major changes can be easily seen on X-ray along with a reduction in the natural joint space.

Secondary osteoarthritis occurs where there is a proven predisposing cause resulting in altered joint pathology. Trauma, especially fractures, involving the articular surfaces of a joint often result in arthritis, as do 'orthopaedic' conditions such as Perthes' disease and congenital dislocation of the hip.

Rheumatoid arthritis

Rheumatoid arthritis is essentially an inflammatory condition of the synovial membrane which affects approximately 1.5 million people in the UK (Hickling and Golding, 1984). The synovitis typically has a symmetrical distribution affecting mainly the metocarpal, phalangeal, proximal interphalangeal and metatarsophalangeal joints. It may also have extra-articular manifestations such as Sjögren's syndrome (dry eyes and mouth), pericarditis and anaemia.

20 MOBILITY

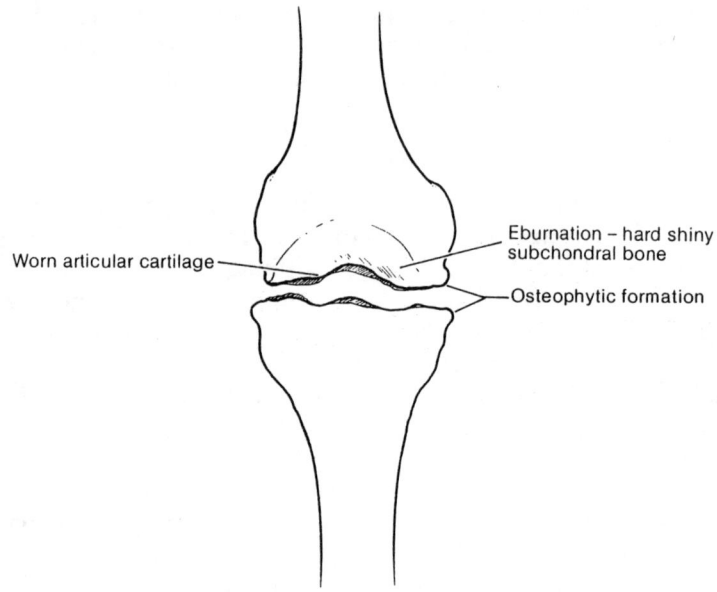

Fig. 2.8 *The joint changes which occur in osteoarthritis*

In the early stages of the disease, a 'pannus' of granulation tissue forms across the synovial joint leading to the production of digestive enzymes which destroy the articular cartilage. The pannus eventually burrows down and erodes the subchondral bone, leaving the joint completely disrupted (see Fig. 2.9). The synovium becomes totally lost and replaced by fibrous tissue. This leads to the contracture of the joint capsule, and frequently the subluxation of the joint. Any synovial tissue can be affected in this way but that found in the tendon sheaths of the hands is especially vulnerable, giving rise to the typical deformities of rheumatoid arthritis (see Fig. 2.10).

The cause of rheumatoid arthritis has been the subject of much discussion over the last 20 years during which time theories such as bacterial or viral origins have been put forward. The aetiology is almost certainly multifactorial in a genetically predisposed individual.

Rheumatoid arthritis has a typically remitting and relapsing course but, unfortunately, the damage to joints while the

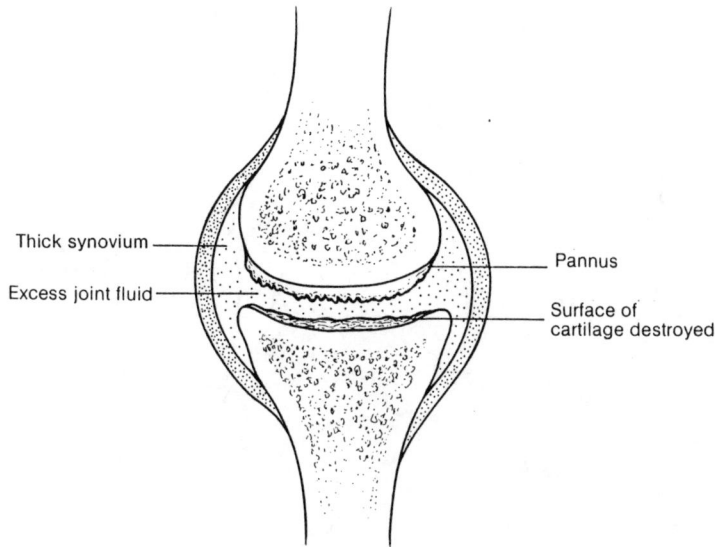

Fig. 2.9 *The major joint changes which occur in rheumatoid arthritis*

disease is active is permanent. This can lead to gross deformity and disability even when the disease is 'burnt out'. The high level of disease activity in the acute phase often leads to hospital admission of the patient for complete rest to minimize joint damage.

Having examined reasons why an individual may become immobile, we will now consider some of the various effects this produces.

THE MAJOR SIDE-EFFECTS OF IMMOBILITY

In their paper on kinetic nursing of the immobilized patient, Millazo and Resh (1982) list 11 major complications of immobilization in a patient with a complete transection of the spinal cord at C5 level. These include the physical problems of pulmonary congestion, urinary tract infection and large pressure sores, together with the psychological problems of

22 MOBILITY

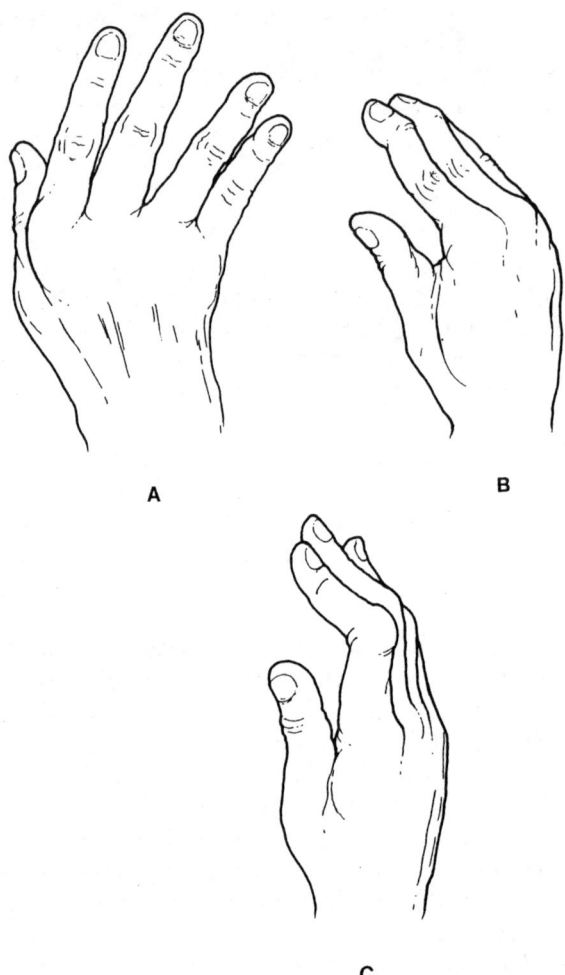

Fig. 2.10 *Typical deformities in the hand of a patient with rheumatoid arthritis*
(a) ulnar deviation of the fingers
(b) swan neck deformities
(c) boutonnière finger deformities

depression and hostility due to poor self-image. In her paper on the physical effects of immobilization, Lentz (1981) suggests that the natural state of the body is that of movement. If the ability to move is reduced, even for two or three days, significant physiological changes can take place.

Pressure sores

These have been the subject of much research and some of the findings will be discussed in detail in later chapters. The ulcer or sore is usually the result of several predisposing factors, but the two most common are external forces on the skin and the internal susceptibility of the skin to breakdown (Barton and Barton, 1981).

The external forces most frequently found are continuous friction against the skin by rough, often damp sheets (this dampness is most likely to be due to the combination of fluid loss through the skin which cannot escape because of waterproof mattress covers), and the pressure of skin and soft tissue over bone.

The skin is composed of a superficial layer, the epidermis, and a deeper vascular layer, the dermis. To survive, the skin, like any other tissues, is dependent on an adequate supply of oxygenated blood. If the dermis is compressed to a pressure greater than 32 mmHg (the arteriole pressure), the area involved will become avascular and eventually necrotic. The time required for irretrievable skin breakdown to occur has been well investigated, and the consensus appears to be that a pressure over 32 mmHg on the skin for 1.5–2 hours can lead to avascular necrosis.

Other predisposing factors in the formation of pressure sores include oedema in the area under pressure making the blood vessels more susceptible to compression (Hickey, 1981), and an altered neurological state in the patient. Individuals with a neurological deficit may be especially at risk due to a lack of skin sensation or inability to move at will.

Deep vein thrombosis

A blood clot formed within the circulation is termed a thrombus. If it forms within the deep veins (of the legs or

24 MOBILITY

pelvis), it is called a deep vein thrombosis. The main danger is that it will become detached and move with the circulation through the right atrium and ventricle to lodge in a branch of the pulmonary artery (pulmonary embolus). If it is large, it will prevent emptying of the right heart, and circulatory failure will quickly result.

In the normal course of events, the return of blood to the heart is aided by the changes in pressure round the veins. In the thoracic and abdominal cavity, this is provided by diaphragmatic movements acting on the venae cavae. In the limbs, the contraction and relaxation of local muscles squeeze each segment of vein and, because of the venous valve system, blood is forced up towards the heart (see Fig. 2.11). This

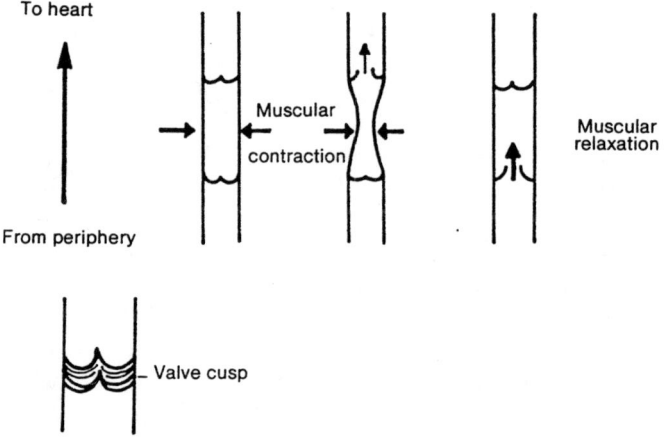

Fig. 2.11 *Diagram to show the muscle pump aiding return of blood to the heart*

phenomenon is known as the 'muscle pump' and is much reduced by immobility. With the decreased blood flow, there is a pooling of blood in the leg veins and an increased incidence of thrombus formation. Other contributing factors may be raised blood viscosity due to electrolyte imbalance, or the higher rate of platelet agglutination associated with surgical and accidental trauma.

Pulmonary congestion

Gas exchange of oxygen and carbon dioxide takes place in the lungs within the alveoli. Gases move from a high to a low concentration via a membrane separating the pulmonary capillaries and the alveolar space (see Fig. 2.12). The inner

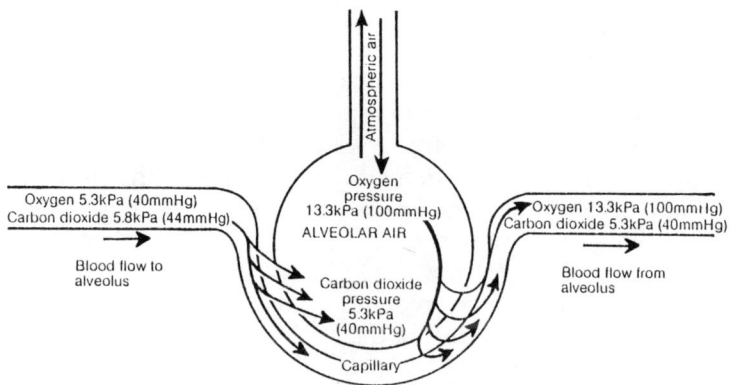

Fig. 2.12 *Diagram to show the gaseous exchange which occurs in the alveoli*

surfaces of the alveoli are covered with a film of surfactant which reduces surface tension and prevents collapse of the air sacs on expiration. Immobility often results in a reduction of surfactant which therefore predisposes to collapse of the alveoli and consequently to reduced lung expansion.

The respiratory tract is lined by ciliated mucous membrane which produces a slightly sticky mucus to act as a protective waterproof barrier. In the immobile patient, chest expansion is reduced by the general muscular inactivity, and there is a reduction in the dilatation of the bronchioles and alveoli. The combined result is the formation of plugs of thick, tenacious mucus at the end of the bronchial tree which prevent gaseous exchange, are very difficult to expectorate and provide an ideal medium for bacterial growth.

The combination of reduced lung expansion, accumulation of secretions and increased likelihood of chest infections, will clearly have serious effects on the patient's respiratory status.

Urinary stasis and infection

With many other constituents, the composition of urine includes several minerals, for example, calcium, oxalate, phosphate and xanthine. In the immobile patient, there is a greater than usual loss of calcium from bone due to a reduction of collagen in which calcium is normally deposited. This results in high blood calcium levels and a raised concentration of calcium in the urine. As a consequence, renal calculi may form and may become large enough to damage the substance of the kidney or block the flow of urine from the kidney in the ureter. If this happens bacteria may flourish in the stagnant urine and cause a kidney infection.

A further reason why individuals with a mobility problem are more likely to develop urinary tract infections involves the use of long-term catheterization. Faecal incontinence and inadequate cleaning of the perianal area are also predisposing factors, particularly in females where the short urethra provides easy access for pathogenic organisms (especially *Escherichia coli*).

Muscle wasting

Skeletal muscle mass is maintained by stress – without it, there is a decrease in mass and strength, and therefore in work capacity. A muscle tension of one third of the maximum capacity is required on a daily basis to maintain normal muscle bulk. Inactivity results in muscle atrophy and a decrease in muscle blood supply. This leads to decreased endurance and rapid fatigue; the individual becomes less active and further atrophy occurs.

Joint contractures

Joints which are left immobile soon become stiff as a result of increased density of the connective tissue surrounding the joint, particularly in the tendons and ligaments. The increase in density is due to failure to keep the lattice work structure of connective tissue stretched open. The initial stages of a contracture have been documented as developing within 36 hours (Schoen, 1986) and will continue to develop unless the joint is put through a range of passive movements at regular intervals.

Depression and boredom

When an individual's status changes from being active and independent to inactive and dependent, the ability to interact with others and the environment also changes. He or she may no longer care about basic needs and come to rely on others. Surroundings may also have altered from that of home and family to an institution and strangers. Behaviour learned in the past is suddenly of no use and, as well as the necessary physical readjustments, he or she need to see themselves in a new role. In twentieth century life, independence is a highly prized commodity and dependence to be avoided at all costs – hence the cry 'I don't want to be a burden to anyone' so frequently quoted, be it from the elderly or the handicapped. In a child, dependence is naturally accepted, and a handicapped child accepted almost as easily. However, an adult displaying child-like dependency has become someone to be pitied, ridiculed and stigmatized (Goffman, 1963).

In her work on depression and the immobilized patient, McCann (1979) suggests that although most nurses would agree that many immobile patients become depressed at some point, little thought has gone into why this should be or the best way to care for such patients. She also states that it is usually only when a patient's behaviour becomes agitated enough to disrupt the ward routine that specialist help is arranged.

If loss leads to grieving, then loss of mobility should produce a similar effect. When a loved one is lost, the various stages of the grieving process have to be experienced; similarly, when a part of the body is lost, be it a limb or an organ, a similar process has to be endured. If an individual sees loss of mobility as losing part of their identity, being no longer a 'whole person', he or she will need help to grieve and to work through feelings of anger, frustration and bereavement.

SUMMARY

Having considered three of the principle causes of immobility; damage to the nervous system, muscles and joints and the adverse side effects such immobility produces, it remains to point out the implications for nursing. Patients deserve to receive and the U.K.C.C. expects that they should receive individualized patient care based on a thorough assessment of their problems. Nursing care should therefore be relevant and based on a logical problem solving approach with rationales underpinning actions. The next chapter will take us down this road. It is sufficient to say at this stage that there is no place in modern nursing for rituals and traditions that have long since lost whatever relevance they once had.

References

Barton A., Barton M. (1981). The medical management of pressure sores. *Queen's Nurse Journal*, 16 (7), 148–149, 157.

Goffman E. (1963). *London Stigma*. Middlesex, England: Penguin Books.

Hickey J. (1981). *The Clinical Practice of Neurological and Neurosurgical Nursing*. Philadelphia: Lippincott.

Hickling P., Golding J. (1984). *An Outline of Rheumatology*. Bristol: Wright.

Lentz M. (1982). Selected aspects of deconditioning secondary to immobilization. *Nursing Clinics of North America*, 16 (4), 729–737.

Leonard B.J. (1972). Body image changes in chronic illness. *Nursing Clinics of North America*, 687–695.

Macleod J., ed. (1977-8). *Davidson's Principles and Practice of Medicine* 15th ed. Edinburgh: Churchill Livingstone.

McCann V.J. (1979). The prevention of Depression in the Immobile Patient. *Official Journal of the Orthopaedic Nurses Association*, November vol. 6, 433–438.

Millazo V., Resh C. (1982). Kinetic nursing – a new approach to the problems of immobilisation. *Journal of Neurosurgical Nursing*, 14, (3), 120–123.

Schoen D. (1986). *The Nursing Process in Orthopaedics*. Connecticut: Appleton-Century-Croft.

Wright V., Haslock L. (1984). *Rheumatism for Nurses and Remedial Therapists*. London: Heinemann.

Bibliography

Jones-Walton P. (1984). Orthopaedic health promotion; injury and disability prevention. *Orthopaedic Nursing*, 3 (6), 35–41.

Lowery B., Jacobsen B., Murphy B. (1983). An exploratory investigation of causal thinking of arthritics. *Nursing Research*, 32 (3), 157–162.
McNaught A.B., Callander R. (1975). *Edinburgh Illustrated Physiology* 3rd edn. Edinburgh: Churchill Livingstone.
Roddie I., Wallace W. (1975). *The Physiology of Disease*. London: Lloyd Luke.
Spector W.G. (1980). *An Introduction to General Pathology*. Edinburgh: Churchill Livingstone.
Versluysen M. (1985). Pressure sores in the elderly. *Journal of Bone and Joint Surgery*, 67–B (1) 10–13.
Wittert D., Barden R. (1985). Deep vein thrombosis, pulmonary embolism and prophylaxis in the orthopaedic patient. *Orthopaedic Nursing*, 5 (4), 27–32.

3
Nursing care and the assessment of immobility

The need for nurses formally to assess individual patients is a slowly evolving belief which was brought to light by the introduction of the nursing process in the early 1970s (although its history goes back to the 1950s in the USA).

While in America, nurses cling to the medical tradition of making a diagnosis – called appropriately a nursing diagnosis – in this country, nurses assess a patient and formulate patient-centred goals. The first two pages of the nursing process involve assessing the patient and planning care, which should then be followed by implementation and evaluation of that care. This systematic way of organizing the care of patients has been a controversial issue which nurses have spent many hours debating, contrasting the traditional task-centred approach to this individualized planning method. A further development over the last few years has been the use of nursing models which set out a philosophy of care. So far, most work in this field has been American.

Some clinical nurses have tried using these models and, fortunately, have found that as a result they have been able to assess their patients more comprehensively and plan care on a logical and holistic basis. By using a nursing model, nurses are putting years of experience at the disposal of less experienced staff.

Chapman (1985) describes a model as a representation of reality and uses the familiar map of the London Underground as an example. This map shows the relationship of the various 'lines' to each other and the order in which the stations occur, and allows strangers to travel knowing that they will reach their destination. However, the map is nothing like the real underground railway. Similarly, a nursing model acts as a guide. It will show the nurse in which direction to aim the care to be given.

Riehl and Roy (1980) have spoken more specifically of a model as a conceptual representation of reality. They suggest that all models, as they develop, demonstrate three essential parts:
1. The goal of the nursing care
2. A concept of the patient as an individual
3. The manner of the nursing intervention.

In considering the problems of mobility we will look at three well known models to see how they can offer a good patient assessment that opens the door to effective care. The reader should remember that a model attempts to answer the fundamental problem of what nursing is, while the nursing process follows on from this as the logical way to deliver nursing care.

ROY'S ADAPTATION MODEL

In introducing her nursing model, Roy makes the assumption that man is a bio-psycho-social being (Rambo, 1984). She suggests that these three elements are in a state of constant interaction both within the individual and with the world outside. In health, Roy sees the person as adapting successfully in these three areas to various stimuli to maintain a balance known as homeostasis. In this, Roy has based a lot of her work on Helson's study of psychological adaptation (1964). An important point which should be made is that this state of homeostasis is an individual state and reinforces the concept of care being individualized. The whole essence of Roy's model appears to be an individual's ability to adapt to various stimuli. Roy describes three types of stimuli:
1. Focal stimuli – those which immediately affect a person, e.g. joint pain.
2. Contextual stimuli – those which affect the person's environment, e.g. the toilet is a long way from the bed.
3. Residual stimuli – beliefs and attitudes which affect the

manner of adaptation, e.g. pain should be endured and it is wrong to ask for pain relief.

Roy divides a person's needs for adaptation into four main areas which she calls modes. They are as follows:
1. *Physiological* – (a) Exercise and rest
   (b) Nutrition
   (c) Elimination
   (d) Oxygen and circulation
   (e) Regulation, e.g. the nervous system and endocrine system.
2. *Self-concept* – the way in which individuals perceive themselves, both physically and mentally.
3. *Role function* – the various roles we all play in life.
4. *Interdependence* – most people move along a continuum between dependence and independence at various stages of their life; patients, too, can often be seen to be moving from dependence on admission to independence on discharge.

Roy's model also divides assessment into two stages – first and second level assessments. The first level assessment describes the patient's behaviour in each of the four modes. In the second level assessment, we pick out maladaptive or problem behaviour and try to identify its causes (i.e. the stimuli).

When using Roy's model to assess a patient with a mobility problem, a whole concept of care is introduced which looks way beyond the 'broken leg in bed four'. We are now looking at the way the patient sees himself or herself in the present predicament, i.e. no longer as a fit, whole person but one whose behaviour must adapt to being ill and dependent. As the role may now have altered from one of active provider to that of passive receiver, the sense of failure may affect the patient's attitude towards recovery time, ability to recover at all and position in the family when he or she eventually is able to return home.

The patient's ability to adapt in the interdependency mode may depend on the ability to identify with the ward situation. The patient may feel that he or she has to fight for the attention of the nurses. As the patient's physical condition improves, he or she may feel a sense of rejection as nurses spend more time with other patients who require more care.

This final point demonstrates the need for assessment to be continuous and not an isolated event performed only when the patient is first admitted.

ROPER'S MODEL OF NURSING

This is probably the most widely used model of nursing in the UK, mainly because of its simplicity and its British origins. The model was originally introduced by Roper in 1976 and later developed by Roper, Logan and Tierney during 1980 to 1983 (Roper et al, 1985).

The basis of this model is the identification of twelve activities of living, some of which encompass activities that are essential for life and some which improve the quality of life. These activities of living bear a striking resemblance to the activities of daily living outlined by Virginia Henderson (1972) and are listed as follows:
1. Maintaining a safe environment
2. Communicating
3. Breathing
4. Controlling body temperature
5. Eating and drinking
6. Eliminating
7. Personal cleansing and dressing
8. Mobilizing
9. Working and playing
10. Expressing sexuality
11. Sleeping
12. Dying

The basic philosophy of Roper's model is the individual's ability to maintain independence in each of these activities of living. Therefore, the age of the individual and place in the life span must be taken into account when considering a patient's position on the dependence/independence continuum.

The advantages of the Roper model lie in its simplicity and its avoidance of American jargon. However, to some extent its simplicity may also be seen as its greatest disadvantage. The model itself does not encourage the user to look further than physical activities; consequently, the patient's psycho-social needs are neglected. The result is a check list of physical problems, but sight of the whole person is lost. However, it does provide a framework on which to base the nursing process and is a starting point in the use of a model of nursing.

OREM'S SELF CARE MODEL

Dorothea Orem is an American nurse theorist who has developed a model of nursing by looking at nursing, nurses and patients and their interrelationship. Orem (1985) has described four concepts on which the model is based. These concepts are:
1. Self care – actions which allow an individual to function with a sense of well-being and social integration.
2. Therapeutic self care demand – the actions required at various times to maintain life and promote health.
3. Self care agency – who carries out self care?
4. Self care deficit – a situation in which the person is unable to meet the demand for self care. This could also include the person's family or 'significant other'.

In their book *Nursing Models for Practice*, Pearson and Vaughan (1986) show these concepts as a pair of scales with demand on one side and ability to meet the demand on the other. Nurses or other agents are required to help meet the self care demand when a deficit can be seen in this balance.

As Roper looked for activities of living which are common to all, so Orem developed her model by looking at self care requisites which are needed to maintain health. These she has termed 'universal self care requisites' and lists them as follows:
1. The maintenance of sufficient intake of air.
2. The maintenance of sufficient intake of water.
3. The maintenance of sufficient intake of food.
4. The provision of care associated with elimination and excretion.
5. The maintenance of a balance between activity and rest.
6. The maintenance of a balance between solitude and social activity.
7. The prevention of hazards to human life, functioning and well-being.

8. The promotion of 'normalcy' within the individual's own frame of reference.

In addition, Orem has considered the need to practise self care in response to developmental needs (e.g. ageing), and also the situation that arises when an individual becomes ill. These are rather awkwardly described as health deviation self care requisites and encompass structure, function and behaviour.

Orem also suggests that the nursing care could be wholly compensatory, partly compensatory or educative/supportive in nature. The amount of compensation provided by the nurse should move from being wholly or partly compensatory to the role of an adviser or teacher. The aim is consequently for the patient progressively to do more and more for himself or herself, while the nurse withdraws from 'acting for' types of care. At this stage, the nurse should assess whether self care will ever be a reasonable goal. Orem also discusses the role of a 'significant other'. This isn't necessarily the next of kin but the person most likely to take over from the nurse as the care agent until the patient is able to continue with self care.

Although use of the Orem model would seem fairly straightforward, it does introduce some new ideas into the organization of nursing care and also about the place of the nurse as the provider of care. Nurses are notorious doers and find it very difficult to stand back to let the patient 'have a go'. An example of this can be seen when teaching patients to dress themselves. It is much quicker to dress patients than to let them do it for themselves, and how nurses can be obsessed with 'getting the work done on time'! Similarly, it is quicker to take patients to the toilet than to walk slowly to the toilet beside them. However, when using Orem as a basis for assessing, planning, implementing and evaluating care, the ultimate goal of the patient being self caring is central from the time of admission.

By using Orem as a framework of nursing care in some of the following chapters, its advantages can be seen, but it has to be acknowledged that there are disadvantages. Nurses' traditional attitudes have been already mentioned, but what of the patient? Many patients, when they are admitted to hospital, are more than willing to let the nursing staff take over their care. They simply do not seem to want to know about the goals or the way in which their care is planned. This apparent lack of interest will be discussed in more detail — both the reasons for it and the way nurses can deal with it. It should be said that patients who are apparently neglecting themselves, or not attempting to practise self care, are still 'legitimate' patients within Orem's philosophy. Their problem is a self care deficit of motivation and possibly knowledge.

ASSESSMENT AND MOBILITY

It is not the purpose of this book to elaborate on the general principles of assessing patients in the clinical area. Many books on the nursing process will discuss the subject at great length, and the reader is directed to them for further information.

However, the specific area of mobility and how it is assessed must be explored. Too frequently, a patient's mobility is given a token assessment simply on the lines of whether or not he or she can walk. As explained in the first chapter, the whole concept of mobility is much greater than that and deserves much greater consideration.

Immobility and the nursing model

Whatever model of nursing is being used, the patient's mobility is almost always one of the areas for consideration. Thus, in Roper's model, mobility is listed as one of the activities of living. However, it should be realized that consideration must also be given to the patient's mobility in several other activities of living, such as personal cleansing and dressing, eliminating and expressing sexuality.

Considering Orem's model, a patient's mobility may be viewed from several different perspectives. As the whole of the model's philosophy is devoted to the patient being self caring, mobility takes on new dimensions. For example, one of the universal self care requisites is the maintenance of sufficient intake of food. That becomes a self care deficit if the patient is unable to walk to the kitchen or use a tin opener because of deformity in her hands due to rheumatoid arthritis. If a patient has mobility problems, it will be seen that there is also a self care deficit in the maintenance of a balance between rest and activity. Elimination and the maintenance of a balance between solitude and social activity, in addition to the promotion of normalcy within the patient's own frame of reference, will all be adversely affected by mobility problems.

When assessing a patient's mobility using Roy's model, all four modes need to be considered. For example in the physiological mode Roy lists exercise and rest as a need, and this would obviously be affected if the patient had a problem with mobility. However, the role function mode would also need to be considered in such a patient, especially in the primary role, i.e. that determined by age and gender. A woman of 35 years who was previously fit and healthy will need help adapting to her role as a relatively immobile sufferer of multiple sclerosis. The nurse also needs to consider how this will affect the patient's self concept and interdependence with others.

Assessing what the patient can do

Whichever model of nursing is used, there must be a normal range of values against which to measure the patient's mobility. The remainder of this chapter will be devoted to assessing the patient under the following headings:

How does immobility affect the patient's life?

Before any formal assessment of a patient's mobility can be made, the nurse must sit and talk to the patient. The information the nurse obtains will fall into areas such as:
1. How the patient's mobility problem affects him or her on a day to day basis.
2. Whether the patient's mobility problem is getting worse.
3. What exactly stops the patient moving as he or she wants to –
    (a) pain
    (b) stiffness – after exercising
               – after resting
    (c) crepitus
    (d) tremor
    (e) lack of muscle reponse

(f) muscle wasting and weakness
(g) limb deformity
(h) lack of motivation or need to move.
4. What walking aids are usually used.
5. How the immobility is viewed by the patient and the family.
6. How the patient thinks mobility can be improved.

Some of these questions may be inappropriate in some instances, but it is essential that the problem is seen from the patient's perspective rather than from the nurse's.

Joint movement

Flexion – towards the body
Extension – away from the body
Adduction – towards the midline
Abduction – away from the midline
Internal rotation – rotated inwards towards the midline
External rotation – rotated outwards away from the midline
Inversion – turned inwards
Eversion – turned outwards
Plantar-flexion – bent forwards
Dorsi-flexion – bent backwards
Palmar-flexion – bent towards the palm
Supination – palm of the hand facing forwards
Pronation – palm of the hand facing backwards

Normal range of movements at major joints

In assessing patients, it is important to compare their actual range of movement with that which is normally possible. This involves the use of a goniometer (see Fig. 3.1). The fixed part of the goniometer is placed along the zero degree line and the centre is placed on the joint to be measured; for example, when measuring the range of movement of the elbow, the zero point is placed on the lateral epicondyle of humerus, the fixed axis aligned with the shaft of humerus and the movable 'arm' aligned with the shaft of radius. The complete range of movement can then be measured.

Shoulder   Flexion–180°   Extension–50°-60°
                 Abduction–120°
                 Horizontal Abduction–180° Horizontal Adduction–45°

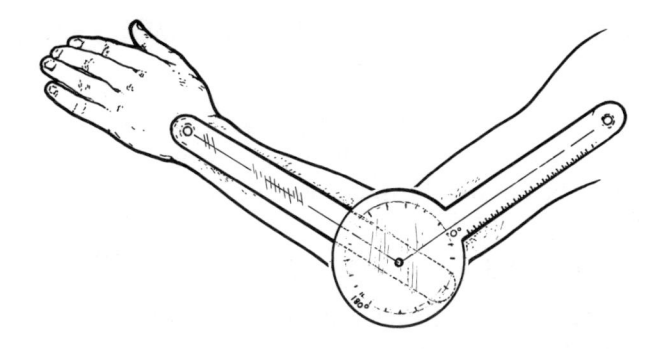

Fig. 3.1 *A goniometer which is used to measure the range of joint movement*

Elbow	Flexion–150°	Extension–0
Forearm	Pronation–90°	Supination–90°
Wrist	Flexion–80°	Extension–70°
	Ulnar Deviation–30°-50°	Radial Deviation–20°
Hip	Flexion–110°-120°	Extension–30°
	Abduction–45°-50°	Adduction–20°-30°
	Internal Rotation–45°	External Rotation–35°
Knee	Flexion–130°	Extension–10°
	Internal Rotation–10°	External Rotation–10°
Ankle	Flexion–20°	Extension–45°-50°
	(dorsi-flexion)	(plantar flexion)
	Inversion–5°	Eversion–5°

Source: Schoen (1986)

Common deformities

In order to describe observed deformities correctly, the following standard descriptions are used:
1. Spinal deformities
   (a) Kyphosis – an increased convex curve on the thoracic spine.
   (b) Lordosis – an increased concave curve of the lumbar spine.
   (c) Scoliosis – a lateral curve of the spine often seen with smaller compensatory curves.
2. Valgus deformities – the distal part of a joint is angulated away from the midline (genu valgus describes 'knock knees').

3. Varus deformities – the distal part of a joint is angulated towards the midline.
4. Eversion – a deformity of the foot in which it is 'turned out' so that excess weight is carried on the medial aspect.
5. Inversion – deformity of the foot in which it is 'turned in' so that excess weight is carried on the lateral aspect.

Assessment of pain

Having considered daily activity and joint function, the nurse must now assess the patient's pain.

In their book on the nursing assessment of pain, Meinhart and McCaffery (1983) suggest that the critical features of pain are:
1. Type
2. Location
3. Severity
4. Duration
5. Precipitating factors.

Of these five features, some are easier to assess than others, and the type of pain and severity of pain have been the subject of much recent research.

Type of pain

In her earlier work, McCaffery (1979) stated that 'pain is what the patient says it is.' It would appear that the words patients use vary so much that it is impossible to generalize about which mean severe pain and which mean less severe pain; for example, is an ache more severe than throbbing pain, and what does the description 'crushing pain' actually mean?

As a result of these difficulties, Gaston-Johansson and Asklund-Gustafsson (1985) looked at the words used to describe pain in their study on developing an instrument for the assessment of pain. The questions they investigated looked at how student nurses rated the differences in intensity of the words 'ache', 'pain' and 'hurt', whether these differences were influenced by the patient's sex or age, and the correlation between the nurse's and the patient's verbal description of the ache associated with rheumatoid arthritis.

To measure the implied severity of the words pain, ache and

hurt, the Visual Analogue Scale (VAS), McGill Pain Questionnaire (MPQ) and a pain, ache, hurt questionnaire were used. The result of this study showed that with VAS there was a significant difference in intensity between the concepts pain, ache and hurt. The MPQ study showed that while there was a high degree of agreement about the term pain, there was a wide variation in interpretation of the term hurt. At the end of this study, Gaston-Johansson and Asklund-Gustafsson suggest ways in which an assessment tool could be developed using this information.

Location of the pain

On the whole, this does not present too much of a problem. An individual's ability to locate the exact point of pain depends on the degree of sensitivity. On the finger tip, two pin pricks can be distinguished from each other at only 3 mm apart, but on the back, the distance will need to be about 50 mm. The patient may need to indicate with a finger exactly where the pain is, but should be able to specify whether it is superficial or deep. However, the issue may be confused by the presence of referred pain or phantom pains after limb amputation.

Severity of the pain

Like the type of pain, severity of pain is extremely difficult to describe and grade as it is a subjective judgement. There have been many attempts to produce an accurate means of measuring the severity of pain. In her study, *The Measurement of Clinical Pain* McGuire (1984) compares the reliability of six pain measuring instruments. These instruments fell into three categories:
1. Scales
   Verbal descriptor scale (a range of words to describe pain)
   Visual analogue scale (marking a point on a line to indicate where between two extremes, the patient's pain is located,
2. Physiological/behavioural measures
   Rating scale for pain (Hanken and McDowell, 1964)
   Pain rating scale (Chambers and Price, 1967)

3. Multi-dimensional measures
   Two-component scale (Johnson 1972, 1973)
   McGill Pain Questionnaire (Melzack 1975)
   Card sort method (Reading and Newton 1978)

In comparing these instruments, McGuire has produced an interesting table which includes ease of understanding and time required for explanation and administering. The author concludes that, whatever the measuring tool chosen, thought must be given to the situation in which it will be used. Only by studying the existing instruments and using them will knowledge be increased and the refining and improving of pain measuring tools be achieved.

Duration of pain

Gaugeing the duration and frequency of pain is extremely difficult, and estimates made both by the nurse and by the patient are notoriously inaccurate. To facilitate the accurate assessment of the duration of pain, the patient may be provided with a pain chart divided into hourly intervals on which to note information such as when the pain started or eased and whether it followed any specific activity, for example, physiotherapy.

Precipating factors

Factors which have been shown to affect the assessment of pain have been listed as follows (Gaston-Johansson and Asklund-Gustafsson, 1985):
1. Attitude
2. Education
3. Experience of health care workers
4. Patient age
5. Cultural background
6. Patient's sex.

From the variety of other factors affecting the assessment of pain, it would appear that the use of a pain measuring instrument is essential if the patient is to receive adequate pain relieving nursing intervention.

Assessment, it must be remembered, is an ongoing situation, not one to be undertaken on the patient's admission and then forgotten. As the nursing interventions are evaluated to ensure their efficiency and relevance, so the patient is reassessed. This is necessary because the patient's problems will change continually.

SUMMARY

Nursing care has to begin with a logical assessment. The models of nursing have been mentioned, each of which has a different approach to assessing the patient's mobility. We may consider how immobility affects the patient's ability to adapt to the stress and demands of life (Roy), the patient's physical independence (Roper) or the patient's ability to practise self care in a wide range of psycho-social as well as physical activities (Orem). Whichever approach is used, we must find out how the patients immobility is affecting their everyday life, what range of movement is possible in the different joints, and finally, how much pain is associated with movement.

References

Chambers W.G., Price G.G. (1967). Influence of the nurse upon effects of analgesics administered. *Nursing Research*, 16, 228–233.

Chapman C. (1985) *Theory of Nursing; Practical Application*. London: Harper and Row.

Gaston-Johansson E., Asklund-Gustafsson M. (1985). A baseline study for the development of an instrument for the assessment of pain. *Journal of Advanced Nursing*, 10, 539–546.

Hanken A., McDowell W. eds (1964). *A study of nurse action in relief of pain*. The Ohio State University School of Nursing, Columbus, Ohio.

Johnson J.E. (1972). Effects of structuring patients' expectations on their reactions to threatening events. *Nursing Research*, 21, 499–504.

Johnson J.E. (1973). Effects of accurate expectations about sensations on the sensory and distress components of pain. *Journal of personality and social psychology*, 27, 261–275.

McCaffery M. (1979). *Nursing Management of the Patient in Pain*. Philadelphia: Lippincott.

McGuire D. (1984). The measurement of clinical pain. *Nursing Research*, 33 (3), 152–156

Meinhart N.T., McCaffery M. (1983). *Pain: a nursing approach to assessment and analysis.* East Norwalk, Connecticut. Appleton-Century-Crofts.

Melzack R. (1975). The McGill pain questionnaire – Major properties and scoring methods. *Pain,* 1, 277–299.

Newton J.R., Reading A.E. (1978). A card sort method of pain assessment. *Journal of Psychosomatic Research,* 24, 119–124.

Orem D. (1985). *Nursing; Concepts and Application.* New York: McGraw-Hill Book Company.

Pearson A., Vaughan B. (1986). *Nursing Models for Practice.* London: Heinemann.

Rambo B. J. (1984). *Adaptation Nursing; Assessment and Intervention.* Colorado: W. B. Saunders.

Reihl J., Roy C. (1980). *Conceptual Models for Nursing Practice.* Connecticut: Appleton-Century-Crofts.

Roper N., Logan W., Tierney A. (1985). *Using a Model of Nursing.* Edinburgh: Churchill Livingstone.

Schoen D. (1986). *The Nursing Process in Orthopaedics.* Connecticut: Appleton-Century-Crofts.

Bibliography

Aggleton P., Chalmers H. (1966). *Nursing Models and the Nursing Process.* London: Nursing Times-Macmillan Books.

Baird S. (1985). Development of a nursing assessment tool to diagnose altered body image in immobilised patients. *Orthopaedic Nursing,* 4 (1), 47–53.

Cooper B., Saarinen-Rahikka H. (1986). Interrelationships of theory, clinical models and research. *Physiotherapy Canada,* 38 (2), 97–100.

Hardy L. (1982). Nursing models and research: A restricting view? *Journal of Advanced Nursing,* 7, 447–451.

Kershaw B., Salvage J. (1986). *Models for Nursing.* London: John Wiley & Son.

Walsh M. (1985). *Accident Emergency Nursing: A New Approach.* London: Heinemann.

Weirner C. (1975). Pain assessment on an orthopaedic ward. *Nursing Outlook,* 23 (8), 508–516.

4
The patient suffering temporary immobilization

Patients may find their whole body or just part of it immobilized on a temporary basis for a variety of reasons, trauma being perhaps the most common. The type of patient can range from a young man who has sustained a fractured shaft of femur which is being treated with traction to an elderly lady with her wrist in plaster after typically sustaining a fracture of the distal radius (Colles' fracture).

If we look beyond trauma, we find examples such as the patient who may have their movement temporarily restricted in order to limit joint damage in response to an acute exacerbation of rheumatoid arthritis. We should look beyond immobility of part of the body to the whole body and remember that any patient going for surgery will be completely immobile during the anaesthetic, and if it is a spinal anaesthetic, the lower half of their body will be relatively immobile for a further 24 hours.

In this chapter, we will therefore review some of the common causes of temporary immobilization and consider the problems this can present for the patient.

TRACTION

This consists of applying a pull to one part of the body against the counter traction of the body weight.

The most common reasons for applying traction include:
1. Reduction of fractures.

46 MOBILITY

2. Maintenance of the position of a fracture following reduction.
3. Resting a joint.
4. Reducing muscle spasm around a joint.
5. Pain relief in patients with low back pain; traction increases the joint space and relieves nerve pressure.
6. Correction of deformity.
7. Pain relief before surgery for a fractured neck of femur.

The two most common ways of applying traction to a limb involve using either the skin or the skeleton itself.

Skin traction

Skin traction is a means of applying a pull to a limb using adhesive or non-adhesive extensions which allow weights to be attached to the skin via a pulley system. Adhesive extensions are not used as frequently now as they once were, with the possible exception of the treatment of children's fractures. Adhesive extensions are strips of special strapping which are applied to either side of the limb (see Fig. 4.1). The weight is

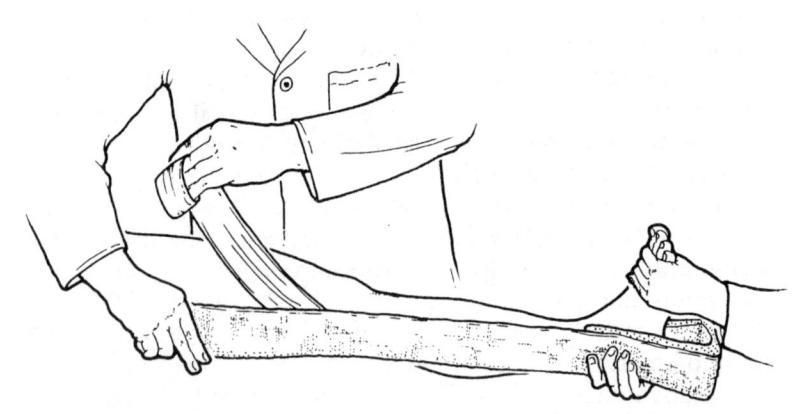

Fig. 4.1 *The application of skin extensions. The limb should be shaved and the lateral and medial aspects sprayed with tincture of benzoin compound before the application of adhesive extensions*

applied to the spreader at the end of the extensions, usually by means of a cord over a pulley. The foot of the bed is then elevated in such a way that the body weight acts as counter traction. Adhesive extensions should always be used where it is imperative that the pull is maintained at all times.

Non-adhesive extensions are strips of specialized rubber with a 'non-slip' backing which are bandaged on to the limb. They are suitable for use when applying Hamilton Russell traction on a patient with a fractured neck of femur or when applying Pugh's traction on a patient with low back pain. It is important that they are applied in such a way that, although the crepe bandage is applied very firmly, the blood supply to the foot is not compromised in any way.

The advantage of skin traction is that it is non-invasive and that an anaesthetic is not required to apply it. The disadvantage is that even the adhesive extensions can slip or peel off, and severe allergic reactions can occur, in which case the extensions have to be removed anyway.

Skeletal traction

To apply traction directly to a bone, as in skeletal traction, a pin must be passed through a bone and left protruding on both sides. The most common form of skeletal traction is found in the treatment of a fractured shaft of femur. A pin is passed through the proximal tibia and a weight applied to it via a stirrup (see Fig. 4.2). Other types of skeletal traction are used in the treatment of fractured tibia when the pin is inserted through the calcaneum, and in fractures of the humerus when a wire is inserted through the olecranon process of the ulna (see Fig. 4.3). The pins used are either a Steinmann's pin or a Denham pin, which is thicker than the Steinmann and has a screw thread half way along to prevent slipping. Kirschner wire is used in the olecranon because of its small diameter.

The advantage of skeletal traction is that a large weight can be applied through it. This is especially useful when trying to overcome the severe muscle spasm of the quadriceps following a fractured shaft of femur. In this case, 6.75–9 kg can be used without any adverse effects. Once the pin is inserted, it

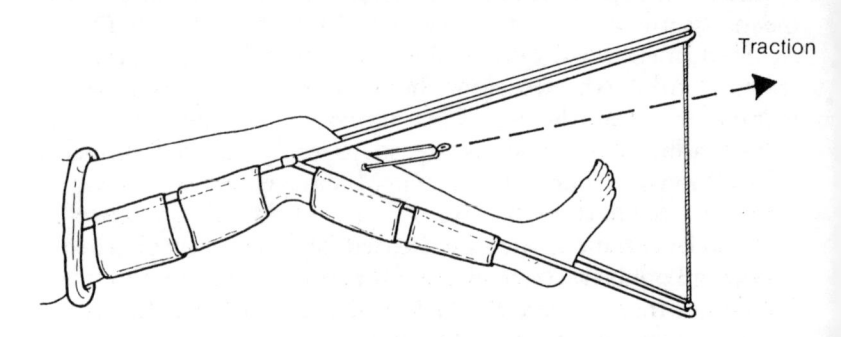

Fig. 4.2 Skeletal traction using a Thomas' splint. Traction is exerted from a pin inserted through the tibia

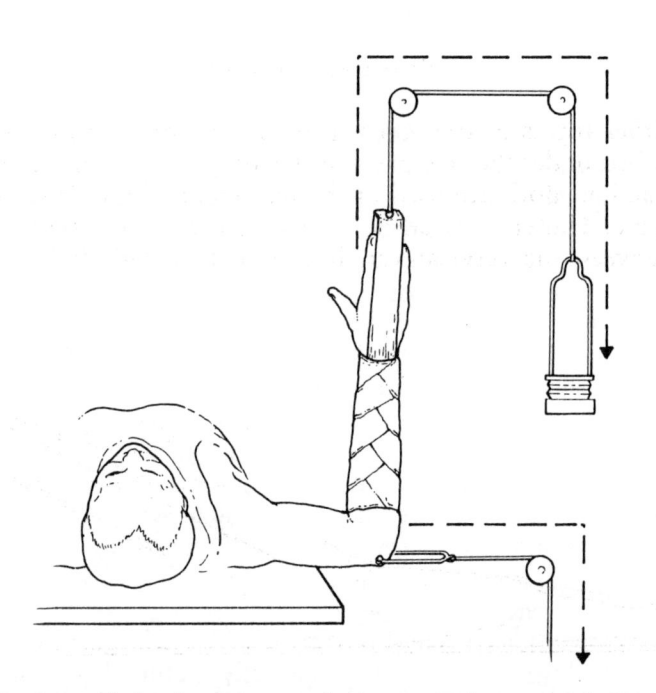

Fig. 4.3 Skeletal traction to the upper limb using Kirschner wire through the olecranon. Note the forearm support and elevation using skin extensions

causes the patient little pain and can be safely left in place for 2–3 months.

The main disadvantage of skeletal traction is that it is an invasive procedure and, therefore, a potential cause of infection. If the bone becomes infected, it can be catastrophic for the patient as osteomyelitis is very difficult to cure. The use of Denham pins has reduced the potential hazard of the pin moving from side to side, thus dragging micro-organisms from the surface of the skin into the bone. Another disadvantage of skeletal traction are found in the very young and in the elderly. In the young, its use is to be discouraged because of the danger of inserting the pin or wire too near to the epiphyseal plate and compromising bone growth. In the elderly, the bone tissue is often porotic and, if the pin is not inserted deeply enough in the tibial shaft, it will splinter the bone and eventually break free.

Other forms of traction

Other forms of traction which cannot conveniently be described under the two previous headings are halter and pelvic traction. Both are used in the treatment of problems of the spine. Halter traction is used to increase the joint spaces between the cervical vertebrae (see Fig. 4.4). It is usually

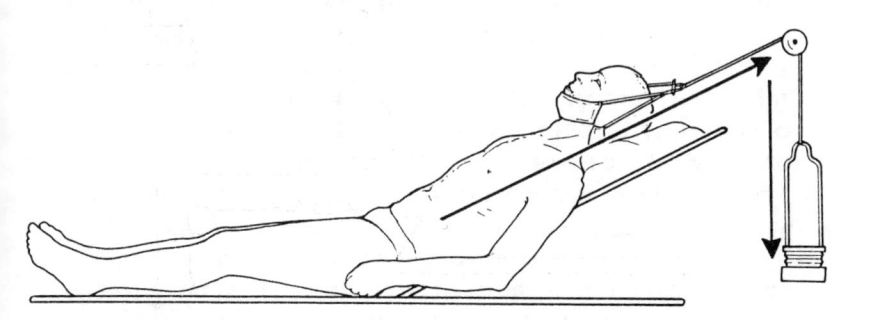

Fig. 4.4 *Halter traction for cervical disc lesions. If the patient is nursed flat, the head of the bed should be raised to allow the body weight to act as counter traction*

applied for 23 hours out of 24 with the patient able to get up for toilet purposes once a day. Pelvic traction is used to increase the joint spaces between the lumbar vertebrae in patients with low back pain. It is an alternative to bilateral Pugh's traction.

Problems associated with the use of traction

Whatever form of traction is used, the problems of temporary immobilization remain much the same. These include:
1. Development of pressure sores.
2. Problems associated with immobility of the legs –
    (a) deep vein thrombosis
    (b) joint stiffness
    (c) inability to use toilet facilities adequately.

Pressure sores

Probably the greatest and certainly the most written about problem of temporary immobilization must be the development of pressure sores – and yet they still occur. It will be understood that this section applies also to all patients who are immobile for whatever reason – not only because they are in traction.

Versluysen (1985) looked at pressure sores in patients on orthopaedic wards following hip surgery. She was able to demonstrate a mean length of stay of 15.9–21.6 days, whereas the mean length of stay for patients in the same ward but who developed pressure sores was 60 days! There has been much research into the development of pressure sores and on the best form of treatment to speed their healing. The conclusion is that, to prevent the development of pressure sores, the total care of the patient is paramount.

For tissues to remain healthy a satisfactory nutritional state must be maintained. A correlation between a protein deficiency and pressure sore development was shown by Moolten (1972) and highlights the need to ensure an adequate protein intake while in hospital. Tissues also need to be hydrated if they are to survive. Elderly patients are especially likely to become dehydrated very quickly as they often keep themselves slightly underhydrated at home to reduce the need to walk to the toilet. These patients may also become dehydrated if they are starved pre-operatively for too long without an intravenous infusion. (This may happen if an operation is cancelled from one day until the next).

Oxygen is another essential requirement for healthy tissues and to prevent tissue necrosis occurring. The nurse must be aware of the ways in which oxygen can be prevented from reaching the skin. These may include poor respiratory function, due either to malposition in bed or a chest infection, cardiac disorder or a blood dyscrasia which inhibits the carriage of oxygen, or a mechanical problem which deprives the local area of oxygenated blood, for example, pressure. We saw in Chapter One that any pressure above the capillary pressure of 32 mmHg will eventually result in skin necrosis. The traditional method of relieving pressure is to turn patients onto their side. This is impossible in patients on traction, and so alternative methods have to be employed. Probably the most common way is to use an 'alternating pressure mattress'. These mattresses are relatively cheap, easily available and fit most hospital beds. They rely on alternative panels (cells) which are electrically inflated in a timed sequence and to a variable pressure. The main disadvantage in the early models was disconnection of the air supply and accidental puncture of the cells. These have been largely overcome, and the major disadvantage now lies with nurses not using the mattresses until the patients develop a sore, or not being vigilant in inspecting susceptible areas for warning signs such as redness of the skin.

Over the last 12 years, the use of sheepskin pads or bootees has greatly increased. Originally, real fleeces were used and Denne (1979) was able to show that these were more effective than synthetic types. Recently developed artificial sheepskins (e.g. Mullipel) are claimed to be much better than the originals, however.

The relationship between incontinence and the development of pressure sores is largely discounted by Torrence (1983). He suggests multifactorial reasons for the findings of Norton (1962) that the incidence of pressure sores in the incontinent patient was 39% compared with 7% amongst continent patients. However, Norton's work would appear to be substantiated by the findings of Lowthian (1985) who looked into the use of incontinence sheets. His results showed that the use of urine retaining incontinence sheets increased the incidence of pressure sores and concluded that the skin's environment was of great importance.

Some patients move in bed more than others, even when they are on traction. Exton-Smith and Sherwin (1961), in a study of elderly patients, showed that those with reduced night-time movements had a significantly higher incidence of pressure sore development. This research has significance for the type of analgesia used in caring for patients while they are on traction. The analgesia must be sufficiently effective to encourage the patient to move around without pain within the confines of the traction. However, especially with an elderly patient, care must be taken that the analgesia is not so effective that the patient spends the majority of the day, as well as the night, asleep.

The use of pillows under the calf to relieve pressure on the heel is decried by many nurses because of the reported increase in deep vein thrombosis in such situations. In their extensive investigation into the causative factors of deep vein thrombosis in orthopaedic patients, Wittert and Barden (1985) list seven risk factors. The positioning of pillows under the calf is not mentioned, but prolonged immobility is! However, in their discussion on the prophylaxis of deep vein thrombosis, they quote work performed by Bergqvist (1983) which showed that regular and rhythmic ankle exercises greatly increase the flow rate in the leg veins. The suggestion is that heels can be cheaply and easily protected by the use of pillows under the calf, but that a programme of ankle exercises should be instituted at the same time. Of course, this would have other advantages as well, for example, prevention of ankle stiffness.

It can be seen that the prevention of pressure sores while a patient is even temporarily immobilized is a major consideration when planning care. Hamilton Russell traction is often used to facilitate nursing and reduce pain in a patient with a fractured neck of femur awaiting surgery. If the patient arrives at theatre with no sign of a break in her skin, the onus is on the theatre staff to ensure that she arrives back on the ward in the same condition. There has been considerable interest lately in the use of the nursing process in theatre and the transfer of care plans to theatre along with the patient's medical notes. In their article on the development of a pressure sore following the use of an orthopaedic traction table, Hughes and Shaw (1985) suggest that the sacral area is at great risk due to the shearing force exerted by the dragging of the pelvis along the operating table, and because of the neglect of pressure area care around the time of surgery when the patient is lying in one position for an excessive time. They conclude by suggesting that pressure sores do develop in the operating theatre and that these are most likely to develop in elderly patients at any point where their skin is in contact with the orthopaedic table. The nursing care of pressure areas is continual and cannot be ignored when something more dramatic is happening. It commences when the patient is first assessed by the nurse and finishes only when the patient is totally self caring.

Problems associated with immobility of the legs

Deep vein thrombosis

This is a well-documented complication of immobility, and the following definitions should help to clarify the relevant terms:
1. Thrombus – a clot in a blood vessel formed from blood constituents.
2. Deep vein thrombosis – a thrombosis in the deep veins of the pelvis and legs, e.g. iliac, popliteal, femoral, posterior tibial and peroneal veins.
3. Pulmonary embolism – embolism of the pulmonary artery or one of its branches, most frequently by detached fragments of thrombus from the leg and pelvic veins.

In the past, pulmonary embolism has been quoted as the leading cause of death following total hip and knee replacement surgery (Sakai and Amstutz, 1976), with mortality figures of 1–2%. Because of these high figures, the cause of deep vein thrombosis has been well investigated. The main area of the research carried out by Wittert and Barden (1985) was in identifying risk factors so that the patients most likely to develop a deep vein thrombosis could be identified and treated prophylactically. Their list of risk factors is:
1. Obesity.

2. History of oedema, pulmonary embolism and deep vein thrombosis.
3. Age – increased risk in patients over the age of 40 years.
4. Prolonged immobility.
5. Patients with blood disorders, heart disease and malignancies.
6. Trauma (accidental and surgical).
7. Contraceptive pills.

As deep vein thrombosis is a life-threatening hazard, the nurse must be aware not only of which patients are at most risk but also of what their main complaints might be.

The patient may complain of pain in the calf which will also be very tender, but many patients have no pain or tenderness at all. The skin in this area may look red, although with a patient on traction that is not always easy to see. The calf may also feel firm and swollen and there may also be swelling over the dorsum of the foot. If the thrombus forms in one of the proximal deep veins such as the iliac vein and occludes it, the whole leg may become swollen and cyanotic. A traditional test for a deep vein thrombosis has been Homans' sign which is positive when dorsi-flexion of the foot produces pain in the calf. However, Barnes (1982) found an approximately 50% inaccuracy when using Homans' sign to diagnose deep vein thrombosis.

In patients who are thought to be at risk of developing a deep vein thrombosis, the prophylactic use of anti-embolic (compression) stockings have been found, in many studies, to be effective. Stockings with graduated compression have been found to be most effective (Bergqvist 1983). The importance of ankle exercises in the prevention of deep vein thrombosis has already been discussed.

The use of anticoagulant medication to prevent a deep vein thrombosis may be indicted if the risk factors are thought to be great enough to warrant it. Although the use of such drugs are relatively safe, they require regular monitoring. The medical staff will check that the patient's clotting times are within the safe limits as bleeding and haematoma formation are potential problems. Nursing staff should be monitoring urine for haematuria, and stools should also be tested daily for occult blood. Any surgical wound should be closely observed for signs of abnormal bleeding. At all times, the nurse should be aware of the location of protamine and vitamin K in case the action of the anticoagulants needs to be reversed urgently. (Protamine is the antidote to heparin, and vitamin K the antidote to warfarin.)

Joint stiffness

Joints which are left in one position inevitably become stiff. If this occurs when the joint is partially flexed, and the patient is unable to extend the joint either actively or passively, a fixed flexion deformity occurs. Changes occur within the microstructure of ligaments and tendons which alter their ability to be stretched.

Contracture of joints may develop within 36 hours after immobility has been enforced (Watson, 1988). Their development is a sad reflection on the nursing care as they are nearly always preventable.

While the patient is immobile, the joints which cannot be moved should be placed in a neutral position and kept there with the use of foot boards, splints and pillows. Those joints which can be moved should be put through a range of movements every 2–4 hours. Where possible, this should be active (performed by the patient), but passive movements are important too, and it is often the nurses' responsibility to ensure that these exercises are performed. Many nurses regard joint movements as the responsibility of the physiotherapists. However, once a programme of exercises has been decided upon by the physiotherapist in conjunction with the nursing staff, putting a joint through a range of movements becomes a 'joint' (!) responsibility. This can often be a test of the team approach to care from the nurses and physiotherapists. After 5 p.m., there is usually only emergency physiotherapy cover, and so it becomes entirely within the nursing care. It is very important that the complication of joint contractures is well documented in the care plan, with adequate nursing interventions to prevent them occurring.

As with any part of nursing care, patient compliance is much improved with patient education. If patients are included in care planning and then encouraged to perform active exercises, the benefits having been explained, this helps them to feel that they have some control over their recovery.

Positive reinforcement for the patient could be provided by a special chart for them to complete when a range of movements has been performed.

Evaluation of the range of active and passive movements possible is essential to ensure that there is no deterioration and that the muscles, ligaments and tendons around a joint have been stretched to their full extent. This is all part of the continual process of assessment discussed earlier.

Inability to use toilet facilities adequately

When the immobile patient is first assessed, the potential problems of urinary retention and constipation must be recognized. For the majority of patients, emptying the bladder and having the bowels open in any circumstances other than the solitude of a locked toilet would appear impossible. From childhood, individuals are taught not to perform these functions while in bed, and it is a difficult feeling to overcome.

Of all the problems of temporary immobilization, this must be one which causes the patient most grief. Their reaction to meeting this problem ranges from those who ask for facilities every 15 minutes in case they wet the bed, to those who just hope it will 'all go away'. It is the nurse's responsibility to make the patients as familiar as possible with the alternatives available, such as commodes, bed-pans, slipper bed-pans, sani-chairs and urinals (both male and female). It should also be explained that it is frequently possible to move the patient and bed into a bathroom to use a bed-pan or commode. The presence of solid walls and a door instead of badly pulled curtains often succeeds in giving the patient the privacy required where all other methods have failed.

For male patients who have to use a urinal and who are on traction, the elevated position of the foot of the bed makes spilling urine difficult to avoid. Occasionally, it may be possible to level the bed but a better solution is to position the patient in such a way that 'run back' is avoided. It is a skill which can be learned, but the patient will need a lot of support and help at first.

Patients on skeletal traction using a Thomas splint often find elimination difficult in the first few days following their injury. Female patients find it difficult to sit on a bed-pan because the ring of the splint gets in the way, especially if it is not high enough into the groin. It is also difficult to pass urine without soiling the leather ring, and this is often the cause of embarrassment. It can be avoided by placing a small piece of polythene over the ring near the vulva so that it drapes into the bed-pan, thus providing a chute for the urine to run down.

Another solution to the problems of elimination while in bed is to ensure that patients have adequate analgesia. If patients equate being lifted or lifting themselves on to a bed-pan with severe pain, they will avoid it as often as possible. This will lead to constipation and to urinary retention which, with good nursing care in the first place, could have been avoided. Patients with a pelvic injury may have a swollen vulva or scrotum which will require even more careful positioning of a urinal or bed-pan. Nurses should be aware that patients with such injuries should have all urine tested for blood in case of trauma to the urinary system.

Patients who have a long leg plaster may find it more comfortable if their leg is elevated on to extra pillows while using a bed-pan. If bilateral long leg plasters are applied, it is important that the patient has extra elevation to enhance comfort and to prevent the back of the plaster breaking down under the pressure of the edge of the bed-pan.

Obviously, other well documented nursing interventions, such as a high fibre diet and a fluid intake of 2–3 litres daily, should be used to avoid complications of elimination.

PLASTER SPLINTS

Plaster of Paris has been used for many years as a cheap but effective way of temporarily immobilizing a limb. Now, more sophisticated materials are being employed with various resin bases which have their own specific properties. Whatever material is used, the problems of immobility that the patient faces are much the same.

The major problem with immobilizing a limb in a splint of any kind is that of neurovascular compromise. Surrounding a limb with a material which becomes hard and unyielding inevitably has problems, as the circumference of any limb rarely remains the same hour by hour. When that limb has been subjected to trauma (either surgical or accidental) or forceful manipulation to reduce a fracture, the soft tissues of the limb will become oedematous, and therefore the circumference of the limb will increase. It is easy to see how the splint, which originally fitted the limb when it was applied, no longer does so.

To overcome this problem, we may use one of two techniques (Bishop, 1989). In the first instance, a full plaster should not be applied to any limb in which there is the remotest chance of swelling occurring. Patients with a new fracture may simply have a back-slab applied to support the limb with a firm cotton bandage over it. This will both supply support and allow for swelling. The following day, when the chance of swelling has receded, the plaster may be completed into a full plaster splint. Alternatively, a full plaster may be applied straight away and then split down one side to allow the plaster to give in response to any swelling. Once the swelling has receded and is not thought likely to return, the plaster should be completed with a plaster bandage.

The patient should always be advised to raise the limb as much as possible; ideally, this should mean higher than the heart. With a cast on the upper limb, the use of a high arm sling (see Fig. 4.5) should keep the forearm at the required level. If the patient is confined to bed, a system of elevating the limb using an intravenous stand and a roller towel or drawer sheet may be employed.

Applying a plaster to the lower limb will require the patient to elevate the leg so that the foot is level with the heart. This may be achieved with pillows, although the nurse must be aware that pillows sink under the weight of a limb and plaster of Paris, and the elevation is easily lost. A more satisfactory method of raising the foot and ankle is the use of a Braun's frame (see Fig. 4.6), although this will reduce the patient's movements around the bed. If a leg with a long leg plaster needs to be raised, a Thomas splint may be used, especially if particularly high elevation is required. In this instance, a Thomas splint will simply need to be suspended from overhead bars with weights balanced against the weight of the patient's leg.

Following the application of a plaster splint, circulatory observations of the distal digits need to be performed regu-

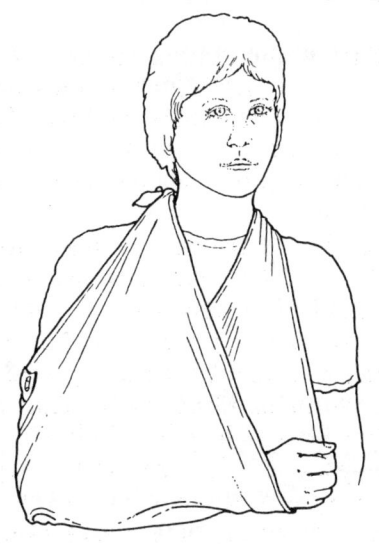

Fig. 4.5 *Full arm sling. Note the position of the fingers in relation to the elbow*

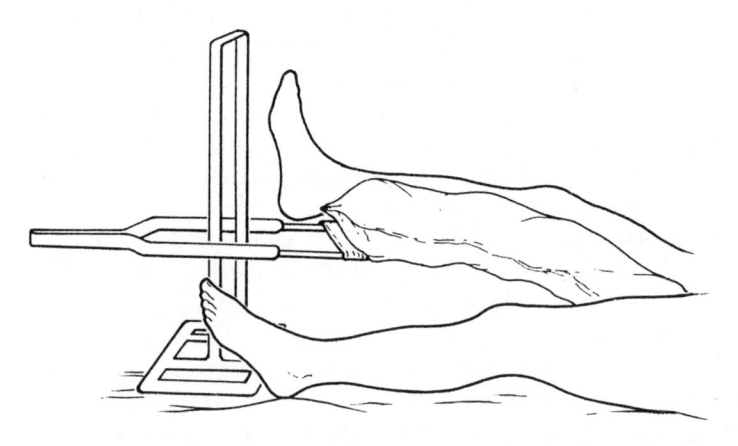

Fig. 4.6 *Elevation of the leg using a Braun's frame. Note that the leg is resting on a pillow with the heel free of pressure*

larly. This should be done by the same nurse to reduce inaccuracies due to the subjectivity of interpreting such observations. While performing these observations, the nurse should first look at the colour of the digit; if it is anything other than a pale pink, it should be noted on the observation chart. While observations of colour may be more difficult with patients of African or Asian origin, observations of sensation, movement and pain remain just as valid.

Perfusion in the finger or toe should be tested to ensure a satisfactory arterial supply. This can be done by pressing a finger nail into the fleshy part of the toe or finger. If the blanched area quickly returns to its usual colour, there is no problem (this also applies to black patients). However, if the finger/toe tip remains white for more than a few seconds, this indicates impaired circulation, the most likely cause of which is that the plaster is too tight. The pressure on the limb must be relieved and therefore the plaster will need to be cut (bivalved) if it is complete or the cotton bandage split down to the skin if it is a back-slab. It should be remembered that a cotton bandage impregnated with dried blood can act much like a tourniquet as it has no stretch. If that has occurred, the bandage should be split down to the skin so that it does not cause any further damage.

At this time, the patient's fingers/toes should be felt to see whether they are warm. White, cold extremities are indicative of ischaemia which needs to be investigated quickly. Besides being due to the cast, this may also be a result of soft tissue swelling within the compartments of the limb. Limb compartments are surrounded by very tough inelastic fascial tissue. In the lower limb there are four compartments – anterior, lateral, superficial and deep posterior. When swelling of the muscle occurs, the fascia is unable to expand and circulation is compromised by pressure within the limb. To overcome this 'compartment syndrome', a fasciotomy may have to be performed in which small cuts are made in the fascia to allow it some 'give' to reduce the tension. This complication can occur very quickly – from hours after the injury to up to six days after the injury (Schoen, 1986).

To complete the observations that must be performed for the first 24 hours following the application of a plaster to a limb, the patient must be asked to move all the digits of the affected limb. Inability to move the digits may be significant, especially if it follows a time when movement was possible. A more important observation is if movement causes any pain in the limb, as this indicates ischaemia of the muscles. If this situation is allowed to continue, patients develop an ischaemic contracture which will result in the irreversible clawing of toes or fingers (see Fig. 4.7).

Whenever a patient complains of tingling or pins and needles in a limb which is in plaster, it must be taken seriously as this may indicate nerve damage due to compression. The appropriate doctor should be notified immediately.

A further complication of immobilizing a limb in a splint is the development of a plaster sore due to the plaster rubbing in a particular spot. In the early stages, the exact position is often difficult to pinpoint and this can make investigating the sore difficult. All complaints of soreness have to be taken seriously, and the usual practice is to cut a window in the cast over the sore area so that the skin can be inspected. The cut out piece of plaster must always be retained and replaced once the skin has been seen and any sore area dressed. Failure to do this may result in an oedematous area bulging into the hole in the plaster, causing deterioration of the sore. However irritating it may be to cut windows in the plaster, it is far better to remove a window unnecessarily than to ignore the patient's complaints. Waiting until the arrival of the smell and stain that typically signify a plaster sore is not good enough! Once the sore has healed, the window can be permanently plastered back into place.

ORTHOTIC BRACING

The use of orthoses has reduced considerably over the last 20 years from a time when every orthopaedic hospital had its own workshop, often employing ex-patients. However, those that are used are much more acceptable than the old fashioned, heavy calipers made from brown leather and steel.

The term 'orthosis' is used for a piece of equipment made to fit to the patient to allow them to function better. It has to be specially prescribed for the individual patient by the doctor with a specific purpose in mind. The main functions of an orthosis are to:
1. Provide stability
2. Overcome weakness
3. Relieve pain
4. Control deformities.

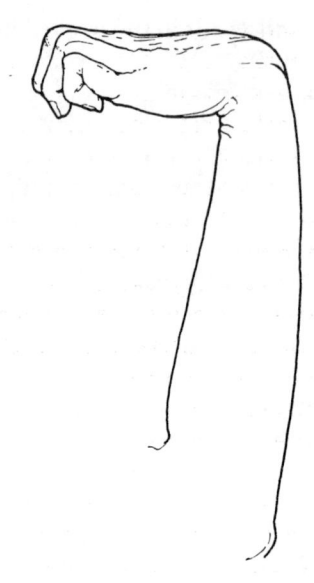

Fig. 4.7 *Volkmann's ischaemic contracture showing typical clawing of the fingers and wrist flexion*

The orthosis may be newly made or it may involve the adaptation of a pre-made splint. It needs to be fitted by the orthotist, and the patient taught to use it. The wide range of orthoses available falls into three main categories:
1. Spinal supports
2. Lower limb orthoses
3. Upper limb orthoses.

The most common orthosis supplied to patients is the spinal belt or corset to support the sacro-iliac region. The support may extend a variable distance above or below the sacro-iliac region. Corsets are deeper than belts and may extend well over the buttocks; they are fastened in the front with straps and buckles. In addition, a fulcrum band extends from the midline at the back to buckle in the front (see Fig. 4.8). The fabric is reinforced with steels which are moulded to fit the contours of the patient's lumbar curve. The combination of the appliance and the steels prevents complete flexion of the spine and reminds the patient to keep the back straight at all times.

Lower limb orthoses are used to provide stability for a

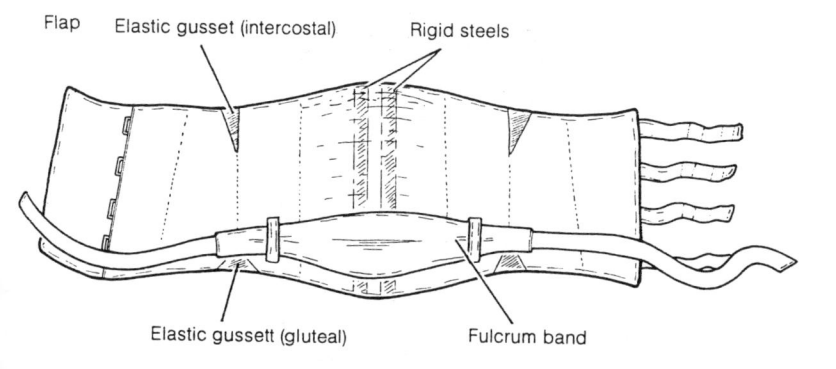

Fig. 4.8 *A lumbosacral corset providing support to the sacroiliac region*

weakened limb and allow the patient to walk. They fall into two main categories:
1. Weight-relieving
2. Non weight-relieving.

In the weight-relieving caliper, the body weight is transmitted through the ischial tuberosity to a padded ring, down metal bars on either side of the leg to the shoe (see Fig. 4.9). However, it should be noted that not all weight is relieved but it is significantly reduced.

Non weight-relieving calipers are very similar but no body weight is supported through the ring. This type of orthosis is used to support a flail (loose) knee joint and prevent it moving abnormally.

Upper limb orthoses are applied mainly to prevent a deformity worsening or to provide support for the wrist while allowing movement of the fingers. Appliances to keep the shoulder adducted between 60–90° may be fitted to a patient before having a repair of the rotator cuff. The splint can be applied immediately postoperatively and worn for 3–5 weeks.

Whatever orthosis is worn, the main principles of care remain the same. The nurse must be familiar with the appliance and the reason for its use so that it can be adequately checked. All the edges must be rounded and have no sharp areas. The patient should be asked if the appliance is comfortable and easy to wear, and the skin inspected under

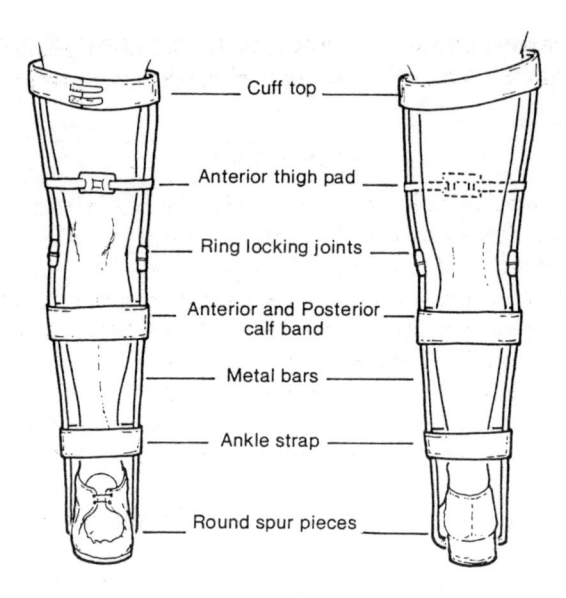

Fig. 4.9 *A weight-relieving caliper. Weight is taken by the ischium of the pelvis resting on the cuff, body weight being taken by metal bars on either side of the leg*

the orthosis for any signs of redness or irritation. Any joints in the appliance should be aligned with the anatomical joints and the range of movement they provide checked to ensure they are correct. All side bars should be contoured to the shape of the limb with plenty of space allowed around boney prominences. If the patient is a child, the side bars should be adjustable to allow for growth.

The patient must be taught to inspect any leather parts of the appliance and keep them in good repair, also to oil all the movable parts regularly and remove any fluff which may accumulate. The patient can also be taught to inspect the skin every night to detect any deterioration.

SPINAL INVESTIGATION AND ANAESTHETICS

Various investigations are performed for patients usually with low back pain to try to detect the exact region of their spine which is affected and also the extent of any damage. For some of these investigations there is specific preparation, but all of them require a time of immobilization after the investigation.

Myelography

This is a procedure in which a contrast dye is introduced into the subarachnoid space. Any pressure on the nerve roots is shown, whether it is caused by a prolapsed disc or tumour. One of two contrast media is commonly used – an oil-based substance (e.g. Myodil), or a water-soluble substance which is most often used in lumbar radiculography.

Patients should be prepared for this procedure by having a sound explanation of what will occur in the X-ray department and the opportunity to ask any relevant questions. Some X-ray departments may suggest starving the patient beforehand in case the patient is very nervous and vomits, but there is no real necessity for this. Particularly anxious patients may need a mild sedative before leaving the ward, and those with severe back pain will require analgesia before the investigation. An open-backed gown should be worn by the patient to allow easy access to the spine.

Approximately 10 ml of cerebrospinal fluid is removed before 3–6 ml of contrast medium is injected, usually between the third and fourth vertebrae with the patient either in the curled left lateral position or sitting erect. The patient is then placed prone on the X-ray table, and the table tilted to allow the dye to flow up and down the subaracnoid space. Many patients find this an alarming part of the procedure and need to be told and retold exactly what is happening.

The dye will collect in the lower part of the spinal cord and gradually be absorbed at the rate of about 1 ml per month. In the USA, some attempt is made to aspirate the dye (as it has a reputation for irritating the meninges) but this is rarely done in the UK.

Following myelography, the patient should be nursed flat for up to 24 hours. The reason for this should be fully explained to the patient as the most common complaint is that of a severe headache which is exacerbated if the head is raised and reduced if the head is lowered. Simple analgesics may be given to reduce the headache. If the headache is severe, frequent neurological observations should be performed to ensure that the patient's level of consciousness is not deteriorating. A high fluid intake should be encouraged, unless the patient is nauseated, and the patient observed for excessive back pain, neck stiffness and pyrexia, which may indicate a developing meningitis. While the patient is lying flat, all the problems of being immobile within the confines of the bed exist and the appropriate nursing interventions will be required.

Lumbar radiculogram

This is similar to myelography except that a water-based substance is used. The significance of this is that the ascent of the contrast medium is to be avoided because it severely irritates the cervical nerve roots and cranial structures, which could result in fitting. Consequently, while in the X-ray department the patient is kept on the trolley with the head elevated to 30–40°. On returning to the ward, the patient's head should be elevated to at least 60°, and some departments recommend that the patient is sat upright. Even if the patient is sitting up, it is suggested that immobility is maintained within the confines of the bed. Once again, the reasons for wanting the patient to remain in this position must be fully explained.

Discography

In this investigation, an intervertebral disc is injected with a radiopaque dye and then X-rayed. Because of the danger of cord injury, this is restricted to the L3–L5 level. It is usually performed when myelography has failed to show any significant abnormality. If any abnormality is shown in the disc, it may be injected with chymopapain which dissolves the nucleus pulposus (chemonucleolysis).

Following discography, the patient should be kept on bedrest for 24–48 hours – usually, the lateral position is the most comfortable. All movements should be restricted to prevent twisting of the spine and log rolling (moving the patient as one unit, like a log) may be used during nursing interventions such as pressure area care and washing.

Spinal anaesthesia

This is frequently performed on patients undergoing surgery below chest level. It is especially useful in patients for whom a general anaesthetic may exacerbate respiratory problems but who will not require a high level of postoperative analgesia. It is a single injection of local anaesthetic, usually given at L3–L4 level, which is introduced into the subarachnoid space and which temporarily affects the transmission of nerve impulses in the spinal nerve roots. Initially, the patient will lose temperature and position sensation, and then quickly loses motor function. The drug will mix with the cerebrospinal fluid and is usually effective for 4–6 hours.

Following the operation, it is important that the nurse remembers that the patient would have lost all feeling in the legs and that his lack of sensation will remain for several hours. Most patients feel very vulnerable at this time and anxious that the sensation and movement will return to their legs. When performing the routine observations, it is important that the nurse attempts to allay patient anxiety by reiterating information given to the patient pre-operatively about the length of time the anaesthetic effects last. During the recovery period, the patient will be unable to change position or feel if the skin is becoming sore. Therefore, part of the nursing care is to ensure that the patient's position is altered frequently and that there are no objects in the bed which could harm the lower limbs by continued pressure.

Lack of sensation will mean that the patient cannot experience any feeling of fullness in his bladder, and the nurse's observation for any distension will be necessary. The patient will also be unable to lift themselves onto a bed-pan or feel when the urinal is correctly positioned, and therefore will require assistance with micturition.

The foot of the bed may be raised as these patients can be hypotensive due to blocking of the sympathetic pathway causing dilatation of the arterioles. Accurate recording of the patient's blood pressure at 15 minute intervals must be continued from the recovery area onto the ward. The bed elevation should remain until the patient regains all feeling and movement in the limbs.

One of the most common complaints following a spinal or

epidural anaesthetic is severe headache. This has decreased over the last few years with the greater use of fine-bore needles which reduce the leakage of cerebrospinal fluid. Patients who complain of severe headaches following these anaesthetics should be encouraged to increase their oral fluid intake and given mild analgesia. Lying flat may also help to ease a headache which persists.

Epidural anaesthesia

For this form of anaesthesia drugs are instilled in the epidural space (outside the dura) of the spinal cord (see Fig. 4.10) via a

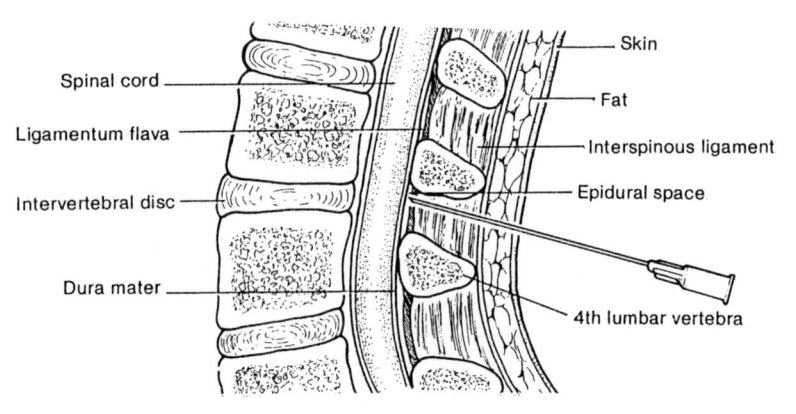

Fig. 4.10 *Injection into the epidural space to induce epidural anaesthesia*

fine cannula which is then taped to the patient's back to allow for further topping-up drug administration. Whether or not the patient loses sensation and motor function will depend on the drugs used. Local anaesthetics will anaesthetize the lower half of the body as in spinal anaesthesia, but opiates such as morphine will work systemically. Consequently, epidurals may be given on their own or with a general anaesthetic as a means of providing very good postoperative analgesia. Patients receiving opiate epidural 'top-ups' are able to be mobile after a few minutes of receiving the drug (within the confines of their surgery). Where a local anaesthetic is used, the nursing interventions remain the same as for a spinal anaesthetic.

Surgery

Following surgery, most patients will experience a period of immobilization, although its duration may vary from 30 minutes to several days. Whatever the surgery performed, patients will have the same sort of problems as those who are immobile due to traction (see page 50). In addition, the following specific problems can be identified, all of which limit mobility:
1. Pain
2. Intravenous infusions
3. Wound drains.

Pain

The control of pain postoperatively is an area in which a multitude of research papers have been published but which is still done very badly. Pain can be controlled to the extent that the patient can move around freely in bed, rather than lying rigidly because even the slightest movement causes agony.

One of the classic investigations of postoperative pain was that undertaken by Hayward (1979), who showed how information and anxiety reduction greatly decrease pain. He also demonstrated differences in attitude towards giving analgesic drugs to male or female patients, and showed that the amount of analgesic which patients receive postoperatively depends much more upon the nurse than on the doctor.

Good, effective pain relief in the postoperative patient is mandatory to avoid the serious complications of immobility, and the reader is strongly advised to follow up Hayward's work.

Intravenous infusions

Only very rarely should the use of an intravenous infusion (IVI) prevent the patient from moving around in bed or around the ward. The main problem is often the patient's concern that the infusion will be pulled out, or that moving any part of the body will affect the infusion. To correct these misconceptions, the nurse should be aware of her role as a provider of information to the patient, and should also try to see the situation from the patient's perspective. Before the patient goes to theatre, the nurse should explain the likelihood of an infusion postoperatively. The exact function of an IVI and how it is achieved could be explained by using a simple diagram and the example of another patient's infusion.

To help the patient feel able to walk about with an IVI, the nurse should ensure that it is secure and unlikely to be pulled out. When the patient starts to be mobile, the nurse should expose the cannula and ensure that it is well secured to the patient's body. This can be done either with elastoplast (provided that the patient is not allergic to it) or the especially designed 'velafix' dressings. The tubing should be free of any tension, and the first 12 inches should be bandaged to the patient to prevent any drag on the cannula. When the patient is dressed in a garment that has a sleeve, the intravenous fluid bag should be threaded through the sleeve before the appropriate arm. To facilitate this, only garments with wide sleeves should be used.

The use of splints for patients with an IVI is often debated. If the cannula has been inserted near a joint where movement may lead to it being dislodged, it would seem appropriate to use a splint. However, it may be that the position of the cannula is such that a splint will not benefit the patient but only make dressing more difficult, and therefore could be omitted.

Although patients with IVIs should be encouraged to be mobile at every opportunity, it cannot be assumed that because they can walk to the bathroom they will be able to walk to wash themselves. Such patients will need assistance with the intravenous stands, which can be extremely cumbersome and rarely seem to run properly on their castors. It should also be explained to the patient that the bandage around the cannula should not get wet as this increases the likelihood of the site becoming infected.

Wound drains

Probably the most common form of wound drain is the 'redivac' drain. As these are usually removed at 48 hours, if not sooner, they do not prevent the patient from being mobile for long. However, it is possible for the patient to be mobile with a redi-vac drain by ingeniously using dressing-gown pockets as receptacles for the bottle, or simply by carrying the bottle in a polythene bag. Care should be taken to ensure that there is no tension on the drain tubing and that the weight of the bottle is well supported.

More sophisticated forms of wound drain, such as underseal drains or those attached to electrical suction, will reduce the patient's ability to be mobile. Once again, the nurse's role as patient educator is essential if the patient is to move within the limits imposed by the drain.

SUMMARY

In this chapter we have looked at the sort of immobility that is associated with short periods of time. The problems associated with traction, plaster of Paris and orthotic braces, and the effects of different types of spinal investigation, anaesthetic and surgery, have all been examined in their turn.

Whether we are using a model of nursing that is directed towards helping the patient to adapt to changes, regain physical independence or practise self care in the full sense of the word, it should be clear that we have to think of the patient as a whole person and assess the problems accordingly. This, of course, is the first step in the nursing process.

The care plan must reflect an awareness by the nurse of the problems that the individual faces, both real and potential, as a result of immobility. Nursing interventions must be carefully planned with the cooperation of the patient if the potential problems are not to become real. It cannot be stressed enough that a full awareness of the patient's perspective is essential, and that only by acquainting the patient with the potential dangers that immobility brings, can cooperation be secured in avoiding possible disaster.

Remember that most of these patients should be able to achieve a high degree of independence once they have overcome their current short-term problem. However, complications such as pressure sores or contractures can seriously delay recovery, while a pulmonary embolism can be fatal. It is up to the nurse to help the patient avoid such potential hazards.

References

Amstidz A., Sakai D.W. (1976). Prevention of thromboembolic phenomena. *Clinical Orthopaedic and Related Research*, **121** 108—119

Barnes R.W. (1982). Current status of non-invasive tests in the diagnosis of venous disease. *Surgical Clinics of North America*, **62** (3), 484–500.

Bergqvist D. (1983). *Postoperative Thromboembolism*. Berlin, Heidelburg, New York: Springer Verlag.

Bishop S. (1989). *Plastering Techniques*. London: Heinemann.

Denne W.A. (1979). An objective assessment of the sheepskins used for decubitus ulcer prophylaxis. *Rheumatology Rehabilitation*, **18**, 23–29.

Exton-Smith A.N., Sherwin R.W. (1961). Prevention of pressure sores: significance of spontaneous bodily movement. *Lancet*, **2**, 1124–1126.

Hayward J. (1979). *Information: A Prescription Against Pain*. London: Royal College of Nurses.

Lowthian P. (1985). A sore point. *Nursing Mirror*, **161**, 9.

Moolten S.E. (1972). Bed sores in the chronically ill patient. *Archive of Physical Medical rehabilitation*, **53**, 430–438.

Norton D. (1962). *Investigation of Geriatric Nursing Problems in Hospital*. London National Corporation for the Care of Old People. Re-issued 1975. Edinburgh: Churchill Livingstone.

Schoen D. (1986). *The Nursing Process in Orthopaedics*. Connecticut: Appleton-Century-Crots.

Shaw J., Hughes A. (1985). Pressure sores and orthopaedic traction tables – yet another skin area to protect. *National Association of Theatre Nurses News*, **22** (9), September, 34–36.

Torrance C. (1983). *Pressure Sore Aetiology, Treatment, Prevention*. London: Croom Helm.

Versulyen M. (1985). Pressure sores in elderly patients. *Journal of Bone and Joint Surgery*, **67B** (1), 10–13.

Wittert D., Barden R. (1985). Deep vein thrombosis, pulmonary embolism and prophylaxis in the orthopaedic patient. *Orthopaedic Nursing*, **4** (4), 27–33.

Bibliography

Chesney N., Chesney M. (1978). *Care of a Patient in Diagnostic Radiography*. Oxford: Blackwell.

Farrell J. (1982). *Illustrated Guide to Orthopaedic Nursing*. Philadelphia: Lippincott.

Goffman E. (1976). *Stigma*. Baltimore: Penguin.

Gould D. (1986). Pressure sore prevention and treatment; an example of nurses' failure to implement research findings. *Journal of Advanced Nursing*, **14** (3), 120–124.

Hickey J. (1986). *Neurological and Neurosurgical Nursing*. Philadelphia: Lippincott.

Millazzo V., Resh C. (1982). Kinetic nursing – a new approach to the problems of immobilisation. *Journal of Neurosurgical Nursing*, **14** (3), 120–124.

Murray D.D., Burke D.C. (1975). *The Handbook of Spinal Cord Medicine*. London: Macmillan.

Norheim C. (1986). Spinal anaesthesia. *Nursing '86 (Westinghouse)*, April, **16**, 42–44.

Royle J., Watson J. ed. (1988). *Watson's Medical and Surgical Nursing and Related Physiology*. London: Balliere Tindall.

Shannon M. (1984). Five famous fallacies about pressure sores. *Nursing '84 (Westinghouse)*, October, **14**, 34–41.

Shergold L. (1986). Epidural and spinal anaesthetics. *Nursing Times*, 2nd July, **82**, 45–46.

Stewart J.M. (1983). *Traction and Orthopaedic Appliances*. Edinburgh: Churchill Livingstone.

5
The patient with permanent immobility of gradual onset

When immobilization becomes permanent, the reason for the immobility becomes less relevant. All individuals who are permanently immobilized have specific needs which will become problems if they are not recognized and met. The range of disability which this term may cover is extensive, from an inability to walk due to a stroke or arthritis, to total paralysis due to a fracture dislocation of the cervical spine.

The care of individuals with a permanent mobility problem should always be aimed at keeping them as independent as possible. Although this may seem common sense now, it is not so long ago that most patients with such a problem were cared for in large institutions. The move into the community has necessitated readjustments both for the patients and for the families. When a member of the family is receiving long-term institutional care, life has to go on for everyone else. Relationships are formed and a way of life adopted that may encompass visiting the hospital once or twice a week as a caring family, but in no way could the family cope, or would they want to cope, with a disabled member in the house. If a family has become used to a wife or husband being permanently cared for in hospital, it can come as a great shock if they are informed by a new, enthusiastic ward sister that, with a lot of hard work, the patient could be discharged home in a 'few' months' time.

When discussing the permanently disabled, the term 'patient' becomes less widely used. This highlights the controversy about the best place to care for those who are permanently disabled. It would appear that most professionals agree that those who are able to should move back into the community from whence they came, whereas those who remain should be cared for in small community homes. Most would agree that the one place that is inappropriate to care for such people is the formal surroundings of a hospital.

Many organizations which care for the disabled actively discourage the use of hospital terminology. As an example, the Cheshire Homes, which care for the young chronic sick throughout the country, have abolished the title of matron and the use of uniforms. Instead, each home has a head of house who is the administrator and a head of care who organizes the care of the residents (including the nursing care).

However, that said, many who are permanently immobile are still cared for in hospital as there is no viable alternative. Unfortunately, the only available beds are often in large institutions which have neither the facilities nor the trained staff to deliver the specialized care needed.

This chapter will be organized around Orem's self care model as this model lends itself to maximizing patient self care and independence. By looking in turn at the universal and health deviancy self care requisites in an assessment of patient needs, the nursing interventions can be discussed in the three subsystems of wholly compensatory, partially compensatory and educative/supportive (see Chapter Three).

UNIVERSAL SELF CARE REQUISITES

Maintenance of sufficient intake of air

Assessment

A deficit in the patient's ability to maintain a sufficient intake of air could be quickly life-threatening. However, by careful assessment the nurse should be able, in many instances, to plan care around any artificial aid the patient requires to assist in respiration. The assessment is also essential to ensure that any deterioration in the patient's ability to maintain adequate air intake is recognized immediately. Orem (1985), in her explanation of the actions required to meet the self care requisites, includes preserving the integrity of associated anatomical structures and physiological processes. Patients are never static; they are a 'dynamic' force always changing in their ability to meet their self care requisites.

In this assessment, the nurse should start by checking that the airway is clear and then look for any abnormalities in the patient's respiratory pattern, be it in rate, depth or muscle involvement (e.g. the use of abdominal muscles rather than chest muscles, indicating weakening or paralysis of the respiratory muscles). A well-known serious indication that air intake is insufficient is the presence of cyanosis, either in the periphery (i.e. the finger/toe-nail beds) or centrally (i.e. around the mouth and the lips. Less obvious is the development of confusion due to cerebral hypoxia, a common feature of the elderly. Any signs of the development of chest infection should also be sought.

Intervention

Wholly compensatory

Patients requiring assistance with respiration from a mechanical respirator in the long term will have a tracheostomy and will need the associated care. (As the detailed care of a ventilated patient is seen to be outside the remit of this book, the reader is directed to a textbook on the specific care of such patients.)

Caring for such patients may at first appear an awesome task, but by using clear explanations and a keen education programme, others can be involved in the care, and the patient encouraged to accept their help. Orem uses the phrase 'significant others' to describe individuals close to the patient who may be taught to be the providers of care. Although the level of physical self care is often very low in such patients, the ventilated conscious patient often learns how to care for himself, and the nurse should accept the patient's knowledge and direction.

Some of the patients who require such a high degree of assistance may be cared for at home, but the commitment of those caring for them needs to be of the highest order. It is not a task to be taken on lightly nor in the highly emotionally charged early days of the accident/illness/surgery that resulted in the need for assisted ventilation.

Partially compensatory

Many patients who fall into this subsystem of nursing intervention are in a transitory state, either improving from needing wholly compensatory care, or deteriorating permanently or temporarily from being in the educative/supportive subsystem.

Patients with a tracheostomy but maintaining their own ventilation will require regular suction to remove the often viscid secretions from their bronchi. Every stage of this rather frightening process should be explained, and the patient encouraged to participate in the care by attempting to cough at the appropriate time to help remove the secretions. This is a strictly aseptic procedure, with a new catheter used each time, and should be performed as swiftly as possible to prevent the patient becoming hypoxic and exhausted due to the effort of coughing. Some patients will require a short period of high concentration oxygen before and after suctioning to compensate for the hypoxic episode. If the patient requires a tracheostomy for a lengthy period of time, a long-term silver tracheostomy is used as opposed to the short-term plastic variety. The inner tube of the long-term tracheostomy should be kept clean by washing it in saline or, if necessary, soaking in sodium bicarbonate to ensure that any dried secretions are removed.

Breathing exercises should be taught to the patient by the physiotherapist, but it is the nurse's responsibility to ensure these are maintained at the correct time intervals. Patients often have to be re-taught how to breath so that their lungs are inflated to their maximum to help in the prevention of atelectasis and pneumonia. Tipping of the patient and chest percussion and vibration also help to loosen the secretions and facilitates patient expectoration. In patients with a long-term mobility problem, the vigorous treatment of relatively minor chest infections becomes of major importance, as often the chest movement is reduced and the patient's ability to expectorate unaided is limited. Any sputum that changes from the usual colourless, thin fluid to a thick, yellow or even green viscid substance should be collected in a sterile pot and sent to the laboratory for culture and sensitivity. Similarly, any sputum that is blood-streaked should be saved and its cause investigated. The combination of blood-stained sputum and chest pain should be treated seriously as it is highly indicative of a pulmonary embolism.

Continual reinforcement and encouragement to maintain the patient's commitment to deep breathing exercises will be necessary. Involvement of the family and significant others will be beneficial. Here again, we see the nurse acting in the educative and supportive role that Orem describes.

Educative/supportive

Patients should be taught how to position themselves in the bed or the chair to help maintain an adequate intake of oxygen. Often, this means several extra pillows to support them in an upright position. It may also mean that a chair with an upright back, rather than a reclining chair, would be more suitable.

The need to monitor the adequacy of air intake should be explained, as should the importance of recognizing whether performing various activities makes them more breathless than it did previously. Frequently, for such patients, it will not be appropriate to measure their walking distances in metres but to assess their ability to transfer from a chair to the bed or to walk across the room. The problem is often that changes occur so slowly that they are not recognized. One solution is for the patient to have a chart so that there is concrete evidence of what could be achieved on certain dates.

Evaluation

Evidence of a patient's air intake being inadequate will be shown by confusion due to cerebral hypoxia and cyanosis. If the care of the tracheostomy tube, such as suctioning, is inadequate, the patient will cough continually and develop a series of chest infections. Arterial blood gas estimation will be a guide to the oxygen content of the blood and the body's ability to excrete carbon dioxide from the lungs. The patient's ability to maintain mobility without becoming breathless will also be a useful tool in the evaluation.

Maintenance of sufficient intake of fluid

Assessment

Patients who are not receiving sufficient fluid may or may not complain of feeling thirsty. Evidence of dehydration lies in reduction of urine output (oliguria if below 500 ml in 24 hours, anuria if below 250 ml in 24 hours), loss of subcutaneous elasticity, elevated blood urea levels which frequently manifest themselves in confusion, nausea and vomiting, and muscular weakness and twitching. The patient may become chronically constipated due to the lack of normal consistency of the faeces. As dehydration becomes more severe, a pyrexia develops due to lack of evaporation of fluid on the skin, and the patient becomes hypotensive because of the reduction in blood volume.

An immobile patient may not maintain an adequate fluid intake for several reasons not always obvious on a superficial assessment. The act of turning on a tap to fill a kettle with water is taken for granted by most of us. However, a patient with severely deformed hands due to rheumatoid arthritis will have extreme difficulty in applying the required force to move most taps. Similarly, many such patients will find holding a kettle over a sink very painful as it increasingly gains weight on filling. Some patients who are just mobile enough to move around the house will find getting up to move to the kitchen such a painful or frustrating experience that they will not bother. Without realizing what they are doing, they will dehydrate themselves. For patients with problems of control of fine movement delivering fluid to their lips can be difficult, with more liquid spilt on the way than is consumed. Similarly, patients with a sensory deficit around their mouth find drinking difficult. It is just the same as trying to drink before the effect of the local anaesthetic has worn off following a visit to the dentist.

Many patients reduce the number of drinks they have to minimize embarrassment or to reduce the amount of urine they pass. For the patient who has great difficulty in moving to the toilet, who finds using a commode distasteful or who has a problem with dribbling or stress incontinence, reducing urine output will appear of great benefit.

Interventions

Wholly compensatory

The patient who is unable to give himself drinks at all will require either a fine-bore system, which delivers fluid straight to the gut, or will need carers with great patience who will ensure an adequate fluid intake by spending a lot of time giving the patient drinks. Again, in her general description of the actions required to meet the universal self care requisites, Orem (1985) suggests that the pleasurable experiences of drinking should be preserved. Since this is impossible with a fine-bore tube feed, so far as is possible fluid should be given orally in the form of drinks. This will also benefit oral hygiene a great deal. To ensure that the patient is receiving an adequate fluid intake, a fluid balance chart will need to be kept in the first instance until a regular regime of drinks is established.

The use of intravenous fluids should not be required in the patient with a long-term mobility problem. However, in a patient who becomes acutely dehydrated (e.g. due to an acute infection), fluids given in this way might be used in a hospital admission to reverse dehydration quickly and prevent any further deterioration of the patient's condition.

Partially compensatory

The availability of drinking utensils which suit individual patients can make a lot of difference to their ability to give themselves a drink. To many, the introduction on wards of drink machines with plastic cups and holders was seen as a great deterioration of standards. However, to those with severe rheumatoid arthritis in their hands or with a neuromuscular condition which left their hands weak, it was seen as a great innovation. The use of a plastic cup inside a rigid plastic holder with two handles may allow patients to give themselves a drink without feeling 'different' from the rest of the patients. The provision of straws to help individuals drink can be successful, remembering that a lot of strength is needed to suck up the fluid. Patients who are generally weak due to immobility, or who have specific weakness of their intra-abdominal muscles, may find using a straw very difficult.

Educative/supportive

As an educator, the nurse must ensure that the patient understands the importance of drinking and the amount that is required in 24 hours. If the patient has difficulty in learning how much fluid intake is needed, a chart may be used as a guide for spacing out the required fluid intake over the day. This should be in the region of two litres per 24 hours. The term 'push fluids' should not be used in any part of the nursing interventions as it will mean nothing to the patient, is of little if any consequence to the nursing staff, and is impossible to evaluate.

Any help that is required in obtaining the most appropriate utensils should be gained from agencies such as the occupational therapy departments or the appliance departments. Often, charitable organizations associated with certain conditions (such as the Multiple Sclerosis Society) are of great help in suggesting where items may be borrowed, hired or bought.

Evaluation

Ideally, patients should be in positive fluid balance; that is, their intake should exceed their measured output. This takes into account the body's insensible fluid loss of approximately one litre in 24 hours, as well as measurable fluid loss such as urine output. Other signs that the care is not meeting the patient's identified needs are those of developing dehydration despite the nursing inventions. In planning care, goals should always be measurable, therefore the nurse should state the required fluid intake in 24 hours. This helps in evaluating care as the goal can be easily measured. 'Encourage fluids' should not be used as a goal as it is impossible to measure and therefore to evaluate.

Maintenance of sufficient intake of food

Assessment

An immobile patient has finely balanced nutritional needs. On the one hand, the nurse may have to ensure that the patient with loss of the swallowing reflex has an adequate, balanced nutritional intake while on the other hand ensuring that the patient with loss of leg function does not become obese because calorie intake is in excess of the diminished energy requirements.

Patients may be unable to practise self care in terms of nutrition because they:
1. Cannot physically reach the room where the food is kept.
2. Cannot prepare the food for eating.
3. Have unsuitable utensils for their individual use.
4. Find the food presented in such a way that it is inedible.
5. Have an altered swallowing reflex.
6. Lack the necessary knowledge of a good diet.
7. Are unable to get to the shops themselves and are dependent on others; consequently, a great deal of convenience foods may be bought.
8. Suffer social deprivation which impairs their ability to afford a good diet.

Intervention

Wholly compensatory

The use of a fine-bore tube feeding system may be required to ensure that the patient receives an adequate nutritional intake. These tubes are much finer than a nasogastric tube and therefore are less irritant to the patient and less traumatic to insert. When inserting such a tube, a metal introducer is first threaded along the length of the tube to give it some rigidity to ease its passage. The tube is then inserted via a nostril into the oesophagus and then to the stomach. When it is thought to be in the correct place, the introducer is removed and kept for reuse. There is some controversy about how the tube's position may be checked. Some systems have an adaptor so that it is possible to aspirate the tube and test the acidity of the aspirate, hopefully confirming the presence of hydrochloric acid and thus the tube's position in the stomach. With other systems, this is impossible and a chest X-ray is necessary to confirm the position. This is essential if the patient is unconscious with either full or partial loss of the cough reflex as accidental introduction of the tube into the lungs could be disastrous.

The dietician's advice should be sought when this type of

feeding is being used to ensure the appropriate feeding required for each individual patient. Once a regime of feeding is commenced, the patient must be monitored for any vomiting or diarrhoea. The latter is a frequent side-effect of this type of feeding but may be significantly reduced by diluting the feed until the patient's digestive system adjusts to the feed or by trying a feed of different osmolality. This will affect the amount of fluid reabsorption which occurs in the gut.

For some patients, a combination of feeding them during the day with food similar to that given to the rest of the patients, and then 'topping up' over night with tube-feeding, is a happy compromise. This allows the patient to taste and eat the food and to gain some pleasure from it without worrying about the quantity, while also ensuring that their calorific and protein intake is adequate.

Partially compensatory

Feeding is one of the most basic things a nurse can do for a patient and yet it is often performed badly. To sit beside a patient and quietly feed him with interest and the correct quantity of food on the spoon or fork calls for great skill. For some patients, all that is required is that the food is cut up into manageable pieces. Again, the use of specially adapted utensils can make the difference between patients feeding or not feeding themselves.

The use of bibs on adults is degrading. A strategically placed paper napkin (two or three if necessary!) can be quite adequate if the patient is helped sufficiently and sat in as near to an upright position as possible. Nurses should always put themselves in the patient's situation. Being 'spood-fed' in this way can be acutely embarrassing and demoralizing for an adult. Is this why the patient refuses food? This problem should be explored to lessen the patient's embarrassment; perhaps the discrete use of screens around the bed would help.

Educative/supportive

The nurse must ensure that the patient's nutritional intake is correct for the individual. Many people need help to recognize their calorific requirements to prevent them becoming overweight. The problem of constipation, so common in the immobile, can be prevented by an appropriate diet. The nurse has a major role to play in educating the patient and family about healthy eating and to point out that it is not expensive to eat a healthy diet. Whether we want an arthritic patient to lose weight or a patient at risk of pressure sores to have healthy skin, diet is a fundamental requirement.

Evaluation

Whether or not the patient's intake of calories is sufficient can be readily evaluated by their weight. When the care is planned and the nursing goals set, the amount of weight that is to be gained or lost, or the limits within which weight must be maintained, can be easily identified. However, besides this, the patient's reaction to the food must be evaluated, for example, whether they enjoy it and eat it or whether diarrhoea or constipation are problems. Food and eating are highly subjective and the patient must, if at all possible, be able to evaluate them themselves along with the nurses.

Control of excrements

Assessment

Control of the bladder and bowels are behaviours usually learned in childhood and associated with cleanliness and growing up. Therefore, the loss of this function is not only a cause of great physical distress but also of much psychological suffering. For individuals with a permanent mobility problem, simply moving to a toilet may be fraught with difficulties. Even with the use of aids such as a wheelchair or crutches, the distance between the doorway and the toilet may be too great. To compound the problem, there is the difficulty of rearranging clothing, especially for the patient with immobile fingers. For patients whose condition has led to the loss of bowel and bladder control, external devices will have to be used to limit the effects of incontinence (Moody, 1989).

Assessment needs to include the dimensions of patient awareness of the need to micturate, its control and the ease of access to the toilet within the patient's limited mobility.

Manual dexterity and the patients' feelings about their problem are also important aspects of managing micturition.

Bowel function should also be assessed, together with the patient's previous history of diet or constipation. The patient's attitude towards bowel function is of great importance and should be identified during the assessment.

Interventions

Wholly compensatory

For individuals who are totally unable to care for their excrements, the embarrassment they suffer cannot be underestimated. Similarly, it is regarded as one of the most stressful factors for carers trying to cope at home (Shakespeare, 1975). Therefore, it is essential that the problem is met head-on and not avoided. For male patients, the use of a 'urosheath' and a day leg-bag may be the answer. This is a very simple system as long as the sheath can be persuaded to remain in place. The 'conveen' system uses a light adhesive strip to anchor the sheath to the penile shaft. When applied correctly, this works well with few side-effects. If long-term catheterization is being considered, the use of a suprapubic catheter is usually recommended. This may also be used in the short term following spinal cord injuries when the bladder is atonic, to prevent over distension.

Patients with a flaccid anal sphincter due to lower motor neuron injury or disease will require a manual evacuation of faeces on a daily or alternate daily basis. Egerton (1986) suggests the use of plenty of lubricant and the insertion of only one finger to avoid anal trauma, including fissures. Although in the dependent patient, manual evacuations are performed with the patient lying on the bed, where possible they should, eventually, be performed in the toilet, which most patients find more acceptable.

Partially compensatory

Many hospitals who specialize in the long-term care or the rehabilitative care of patients with bowel and bladder problems have a bladder training programme. This is a fairly rigid programme which requires the patient to drink at set intervals throughout the day and attempt to empty their bladder at set times. A residual catheterization is performed after each attempt to void. A residual of 100 ml or less is usually regarded as satisfactory, and the bladder training programme continues. When more than 100 ml of urine remains in the bladder, a catheter should remain in situ and the training programme re-scheduled on another day.

There has been a great increase in recent years in teaching patients to catheterize themselves intermittently. Nursing care, therefore, would quickly move towards the educative system. Obviously, the patient needs good control of the upper limbs to perform self-catheterization but, if it is possible, it ensures that the bladder is emptied regularly, in a convenient place with a much smaller risk of cross infection (Hickey, 1986). Self-catheterization is performed with a short, straight catheter which is removed each time. At first, it is performed every 4–6 hours but later it can be timed to suit the patient's needs. Many patients who have a problem emptying their bladders due to a spinal cord lesion are able to be stimulated to do so by stroking of the thigh, abdomen or genitalia or by anal massage.

Educative/supportive

Patients who have lost anal sphincter control should be taught how to perform their own manual evacuations, if that is possible. Sometimes, a 'significant other' can also be taught how to do it, but both individuals will need a lot of support in the early stages of the education programme. It requires a special relationship either to survive that state of dependency or to overcome the natural repulsion of emptying another's bowel content.

The education of patients in the promotion and maintenance of continence is an area of nursing care with great rewards for the nurse. Many health authorities have an expert in the care of those with a continence problem, and the advice of this specialist should be sought as soon as possible. Incontinence should always be treated in a positive way, and adult patients should never be treated as naughty children if they are found to be in a 'wet state' or if their appliance has leaked. Learning to become continent again takes a lot of positive effort and determination on the part of both the patient and nurse. Relatives will also need to be taught about the reasons for incontinence and the means of overcoming the problem.

Once continence or an adequate system of containing urine output has been achieved, the patient will be able to wear a greater variety of clothes, which will improve their self-image so that they feel much more 'socially acceptable' within the community. This, in turn, will open the world of visiting, shopping and other expeditions to those who were previously house-bound because they were always wet or leaking urine.

Evaluation

The goal of nursing intervention must be that the patient will reach as near a state of continence as possible. If that remains an unrealistic goal, an alternative system of storing the urine must be found. This must be comfortable, simple to manage and above all leakproof so that the patient can develop some confidence in it. The other goal is that the patient will be free of urinary complications such as renal calculi or urinary tract infection. Patients need to be taught about these complications, what causes them and how they can be dealt with. Often, the patient will be able to feel that there is something wrong before any obvious symptoms are apparent.

The effectiveness of a programme of bladder training can be evaluated by careful documentation of incontinent episodes. Such a chart can reveal any pattern of incontinence through the 24 hours of the day and, over a period of a week or two, allow both staff and patient to see how much progress is being made. Similarly, bowel activities should be regularly charted to see how effective the nursing care is in avoiding constipation on the one hand and faecal incontinence on the other. Only by setting patient goals that are measurable can nursing care be evaluated properly. One final point concerns the patients' attitude towards their problem. Not only should this be fully assessed at the start, but it should be the subject of reassessment at regular intervals to see whether the patients are better able to accept their continence problems and how motivated they are to continue with any retraining programme.

Maintenance of a balance between activity and rest

Assessment

Any individual with a permanent mobility problem has an imbalance between activity and rest. The extent of this imbalance will vary considerably from those who are able to move their upper limbs and perform a lot of their daily activities, to those who are confined to bed and totally dependent on others. Immobility restricts not only movement but also the way one individual interacts with another. Independence has to give way to dependence, which holds negative connotations for many people. Independence is a highly prized commodity in our society, remove it and immediately adulthood starts to be replaced by childhood and the whole 'does he take sugar' syndrome. Even when an individual is dependent in only one area of functioning, they are frequently assumed to be dependent in others. For example, an individual who is blind is often shouted at on the assumption that he or she is deaf as well. Seligman (1978) used the term 'learned helplessness' to describe the effect of immobility on an individual. It can lead to feelings of passivity about the patient's surroundings and the influence that the patient may have on them.

Adults who are dependent on others are often 'looked down on' in our society. Little is organized for them in our towns and cities – even the 'disabled toilets' are frequently locked and a special journey has to be made to another venue to obtain the key.

When assessing a patient's ability to move, the nurse will need to work with the physiotherapist who obviously will have a specific interest in this aspect of the patient's care. This is one area where the 'multidisciplinary approach' comes into its own and the responsibilities of the nurse, physiotherapist and occupational therapist overlap. It is important to remember that the assessment calls for a balance between activity and rest, and that too much activity by the 'caring team' will reduce the amount of rest the patient has, which may be

detrimental. When assessing a patient with a permanent mobility problem, the nurse will need to look at:
1. What movement the patient has.
2. Whether or not it is likely to improve at all.
3. How the lack of movement is affecting the patient emotionally/physically.
4. Whether there is a reduction in the amount of rest enjoyed by the patient because of pain, muscle spasm or anxiety.

At this assessment, the physiotherapist will be looking to see what supportive aids might be of use to the patient, such as a spinal brace to aid sitting, and the occupational therapist may be looking at the suitability of various types of wheelchair that could be used in the future, as well as splinting methods to correct deformities or reduce the muscle spasm.

It should be recognized that for patients with a progressive disease, regular detailed assessments can have a profoundly depressing effect (Burford, 1985). This author found that it was more beneficial to concentrate on the changing functional abilities of the patient.

Intervention

Wholly compensatory

Patients who are unable to move at all or whose movement is deteriorating due to a progressive disease, such as motor neuron disease or multiple sclerosis, will need considerable support to compensate for the loss of such a basic activity. While the nursing care will focus on the prevention of physical complications such as we have discussed already, sight should not be lost of the equally important psychological and social problems that will accompany such a condition.

The use of special beds and mattresses for patients with a permanent mobility problem has been the subject of much enquiry. Among the various beds available, the important features are that their height should be easily adjustable, they should have adequate brakes on the front and the rear wheels, and they should provide a firm base for the mattress. Other features may include split bases such as in the Stoke Egerton bed (see Fig. 5.1), which is electronically controlled and facilitates turning the patient from side to side. This bed also

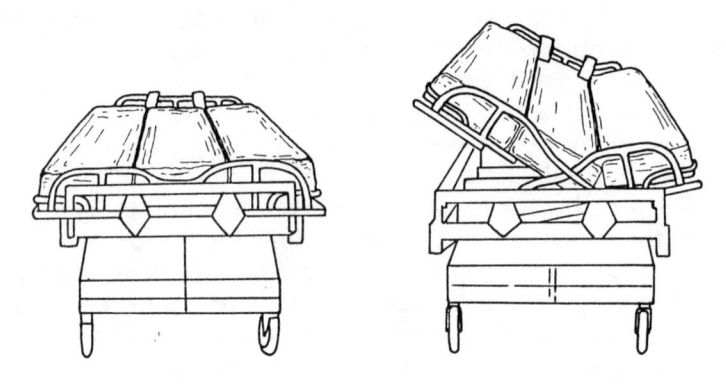

Fig. 5.1 *An electric turning bed*

has the advantage of a wide base so that it can be used for extremely obese patients with safety. A profiling bed, in which the base has three sections that can be individually manoeuvred to change the patient's position (see Fig. 5.2), is

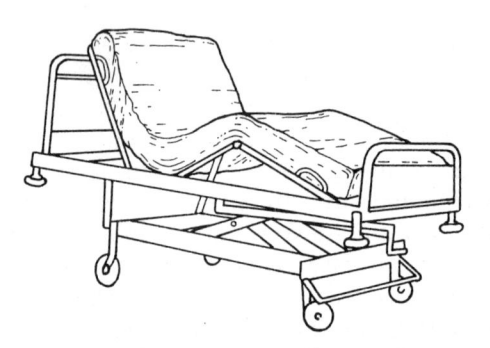

Fig. 5.2 *A profiling bed*

frequently used for those with a spinal injury.

Stryker frames (see Fig. 5.3) were used for patients with spinal injuries as they allowed turning from front to back while maintaining skull traction. They comprise an anterior and posterior shell. When the patient is turned to the prone position, the anterior shell is fixed to the posterior shell and, with the patient sandwiched in the middle, the whole frame is turned by the use of a handle. The posterior shell may then be removed, and the skin washed and inspected. Stryker frames

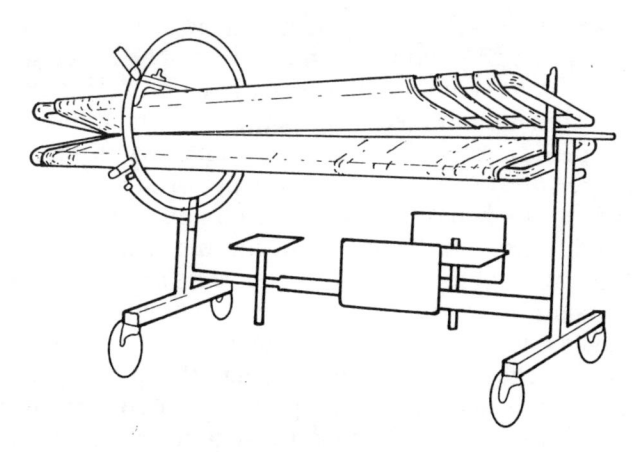

Fig. 5.3 *A Stryker turning frame*

were also used for patients following spinal surgery. Their use is declining as they look quite barbaric and make the patients feel very vulnerable. Probably, their greatest advantage was that they enabled two nurses to turn a totally immobile patient. However, they did require a high degree of skill from the nurses and great trust by the patient in that skill. As their use declines, so does the number of nurses with the necessary expertise to use the frames. Usually, a more acceptable alternative can be found.

Mattresses and mattress covers have been blamed in the past for skin breakdown with a certain justification. The search for a cover which can be washed and is therefore waterproof, which does not wrinkle nor cause pooling of sweat, has been long and hard. Whatever bed or mattress is used, nothing can replace constant vigilance by the nursing staff in the search for 'marking' on the patient's skin. Marking always indicates an unacceptable pressure on the skin and therefore the need for immediate action to relieve that pressure.

As the patient is unable to move certain joints, the need is for regular passive movements to be carried out by the nursing staff. These have been found in some instances to reduce joint pain, preserve joint function and prevent muscle shortening, although there is some controversy about the frequency at which these movements should be carried out. Whenever these passive exercises are performed, it is important that joints are protected and not put under any undue stress.

Nursing interventions which may help to reduce the patient's anxiety and therefore promote rest include encouragement in the contraction and relaxation of whatever muscle groups are still functioning (even the use of facial muscles in this way can be beneficial, although obviously patients with such conditions as arthritis benefit more as they are able to move a greater number of muscles). A nurse's time may be the greatest commodity that can be given to patients, along with encouragement to express their fears and the causes of anxieties. Hickey (1986) suggests that the patient will be helped by involvement with all aspects of care so that a feeling of control is maintained. Long days lying in a hospital bed, or at home, immobile and highly dependent on others, can have a very depressing effect on patients. They may think back to better times before their illness and reflect on their activity then, perhaps working through a grieving process for their lost independence. Nurses should try to imagine how they would react to such a loss of mobility and be aware that psychological support is as important as physical care.

The use of computers has given many immobile individuals the opportunity to have some kind of meaningful recreation, be it playing games, creative writing or involvement with writing programmes that will benefit others. The participation of colleges of further education with computer technology departments to help individual patients has to be encouraged as it has a practical value and also makes the patient feel important. Every effort should be made to give the patient meaningful mental activity to prevent boredom and give some feeling of worth and value. This should extend far beyond the ubiquitous television set and involve family, the occupational therapy department and some creative, imaginative thinking by nursing staff.

Nursing interventions in this subsystem will include helping the patient to be as active as possible. This will mean promoting independence in various activities such as washing, shaving and dressing. It can be a frustrating time for the patient and for the nurse as both parties know that the nurse would perform these activities quicker and probably more efficiently. It may entail the nurse taking the patient to the toilet in a wheelchair and then encouraging the patient to walk back to the bed. The maintenance of residual movement is fundamental in improving the level of activity. The nursing care plan should include a detailed indication of the patient's level of activity so that improvement or deterioration can be measured.

Goals such as 'mobilize gently' are meaningless as they are impossible to measure. The mobility goals that the patient is aiming for must be stated in terms that can be measured such as 'will walk to the day room with a zimmer frame, unaided' or 'will walk 10 yards with the aid of a tripod walking stick'. Dates that are realistic for the achievement of these goals should also be included.

Many patients who are cared for in special units for those with a long-term mobility problem are able to take advantage of the social events organized either by the unit or by charitable organizations. In this respect, such patients have a great advantage over those in a district general hospital, which rarely have such facilities. Care has to be taken by the managers of specialist units to ensure that the individuality of the patient is not ignored. Volunteers may assume that all patients will be grateful for a concert or a trip to the zoo whereas, in fact, they may hate it and yet be in a position where it is difficult to refuse.

Ben-Schlomo and Short (1985) looked at the effect of physical activity on sedentary females and found that those who had partaken in a specific programme to improve their activity gained in feelings of self-esteem and appearance. Similar findings were found by Goldberg and Fitzpatrick (1980). In their paper it was shown that a group in a nursing home who followed a programme of movement therapy had a more positive attitude towards their own ageing and also enjoyed an uplifting of morale.

Patients should not be left to slump in the chair staring at an empty wall. Efforts must be made to provide some form of recreational activity that suits the patient. To help achieve this, relatives and significant others can be enrolled to provide ideas and materials. Active brains trapped in a inactive body become frustrated and demoralized.

The detrimental effects of sleep deprivation are well known. The patients care should therefore include a goal to the effect that they will have a set number of hours sleep per night; however, the actual number and the times between which the patient sleeps should reflect the patients normal sleep patterns as far as possible if we are to practise truly individualized care.

Educative support

The role of the nurse in this subsystem is to provide the patient and the carers or significant others with sufficient knowledge for the patient to remain as self caring as possible for as long as possible. Passive exercises can be taught and performed at home as easily as in hospital, as can care of special beds and pressure areas. For self care to be a viable alternative to institutional care, the patient and significant others will need to know as much as possible about the medical condition and the potential problems that may arise. Patients and family should know about the effect that inactivity could have on them emotionally and how to overcome the problem. Similarly, advice should be given on lifting and transferring the patient from bed to chair or wheelchair. Before such a patient could leave hospital, a training programme will be needed both for the patient and for significant others to enable the transfer from hospital to be as smooth as possible. Very close liaison between hospital and community nurses is essential in the care of the patient before and after discharge.

In this role, the nurse may be seen as the coordinator, ensuring that all aids are available at home. While it is the function of the occupational therapist and social worker to ensure that the family have whatever help is available, both financially and in terms of adaptations to the home, the nurse has the very important role of educating the family about what might be available. If families are unaware of assistance, they will not ask, and so may be deprived of valuable resources.

Evaluation

The efficacy of the nursing interventions can be measured by the prevention of complications of long-term inactivity. Thus, if the care has been right, the patient will remain free of pressure sores, will not develop a deep vein thrombosis and will retain a positive attitude towards the future. For patients whose condition will improve enough for them to have sitting in a wheelchair or even standing in a frame as realistic goals, the prevention of muscle shortening and joint contraction is vital. If contractions occur, the patient will need to undergo tendon lengthening operations.

For patients to have a positive attitude towards themselves and their future, the need for rest is paramount. Sleep deprivation and inadequate rest are detrimental to mental and physical health; consequently, the evaluation stage should include careful monitoring of how many hours sleep the patient manages per night.

Balance between solitude and social activity

Assessment

Most mobile individuals are able to decide when they wish to be on their own and when they require company and to act accordingly. Those with a permanent mobility problem do not have that privilege. They can be lying in bed desperate to talk to someone or sat in a day room, having been wheeled there, listening to someone talking at them and hating every minute of it. As with every other assessment, the nurse must talk at length to the patient to assess the amount of solitude and social activity that the patient expects. Again, it is the 'balance that is right for the patient' that is important, not the nurses opinion of what is right for the patient.

When individuals become immobile, the way they interact with their environment is altered. Because of this, there may be a difficulty when, for example, work colleagues come to visit, as this may remind the patient of their former independent life style. Such thoughts may be too painful for the patient and so they cope by shutting out the past, surprising everyone by demanding that the visitors be banned. The need here is for nursing staff to comply with the patient's wishes in the immediate situation, and then to sit down quietly with the patient later and try to talk through the problem. By getting the patient to verbalize their *real* reason for refusing visitors, a major step has been taken in resolving the difficulty.

Patients who are having problems in adjusting to an altered

self-image may find it easier to relate to children visiting or even the family pet. This may prove to be a slightly less threatening re-introduction to their previous lifestyle. Assessment needs to find out the level of social activity enjoyed by patients before reaching the present state of immobility, as well as their feelings about socialization now.

Intervention

Wholly compensatory

For individuals with a permanent mobility problem, totally depending on others to provide social interaction or ensuring solitude is demeaning. Added to this is the well known problem of ensuring any kind of privacy in hospital. Except in private rooms, which may bring their own problems of loneliness, beds tend to be close enough together for neighbours to overhear conversations. This can be a particular problem for partners who need to have some time together to talk over the more intimate details of their lives. Couples who have been used to an active sex life but which is now curtailed by immobility will find, eventually, that sitting holding hands is not sufficient to meet their needs. The physical and emotional frustration that builds up can cause severe problems which affect not only the couple but also the rest of the family and the nursing staff.

If a couple wish to be intimate together, the patient's bed could be pushed into an empty side ward or even an empty bathroom if there is nowhere else. All that may be required is a room with walls and a door that locks rather than a bed-space surrounded by short curtains. In any case, the nurse should be aware of this aspect of the patient's care to be able to suggest such a solution. Eventually, the help of a professional psychosexual counsellor may be engaged as there are ways of overcoming most of the problems immobility adds to an active sex life. It may be simply a case of a change of position from that which had been practised in the past. For male patients with a neurological condition, the use of a vibrator may stimulate ejaculation or help to initiate and maintain an erection. It will be a time in which both partners require great help and support, but with a positive attitude most problems can be overcome. The important point is recognition of the problem and engaging professional help.

Partially compensatory

Patients who require this level of nursing care to maintain a balance of social interaction and solitude are often in a wheelchair and may or may not require help pushing the chair. In specialist units, trips are often organized for patients in chairs either to the local shops or public house. This leads to nurses being cajoled into acting as their pushers often in off-duty time. The nurse should be aware in this situation of the feelings that can arise within a unit if one patient is seen to be preferred over another. It should be recognized that some nurses get on better with some patients than with others; however, all patients should be treated equally and not just a chosen few given the bonus of a trip out of the hospital.

For those patients who have more serious difficulty adjusting to this balance between socializing and solitude, a visit by a clinical psychologist may be of benefit.

Supportive/educative

Self help specialist support groups can be a great help to patients not only with practical tips but also in providing experiences with similar problems. Patients can often be linked to these groups by the nursing staff and a visit arranged while the patient is still in hospital.

Probably the greatest help the nurse can be in this subsystem is by making the patient aware that any negative thoughts and feelings which might be felt are part of the process of coming to terms with immobility and its problems.

Evaluation

Whether or not the patient achieves this balance between solitude and social activity is only measured by the patient. The nurse may delight in seeing the patient taking part in many ward activities but be unaware that the patient is hating every minute. An informal, open atmosphere in the ward or unit is one that will invite the patient to express any opinions of feelings about organized social occasions.

The involvement of a clinical psychologist or counsellor who is able to run groups within the ward or unit may be an eye-opener for the ward staff. In this situation, it is important that the staff have good support as it can seem threatening for them. The families of patients could also be involved in these meetings. With a skilful leader, many problems can be aired and reduced to a manageable size, even if not solved.

Prevention of hazards to life, functioning and well-being

Assessment

In her explanation of this part of the model, Orem (1985) describes the prevention of hazards as contributing to the maintenance of human integrity and thus to the effective promotion of human functioning. By looking at the promotion of human functioning and development, the potential problems that might arise are anticipated and may be prevented. Orem also explains that it may be a case of removing the hazard itself or removing oneself from the hazard. She suggests that hazards should be looked at in conjunction with the previous parts of the universal self care requisites, i.e. sufficient intake of water, air and food, elimination, the balance between rest and activity, and the balance between solitude and social interaction.

When assessing a patient using this model, the nurse should look at the ways in which a patient's needs may alter to ensure that the nursing care that was suitable has not become a hazard to the patient. The patient's environment should be carefully examined to ensure that it is free from hazards. Nursing care may be directed towards mobilizing the patient, say by assisting with a walk of 10 yards every two hours. However, if the patient is not wearing appropriate footwear or does not understand that nursing assistance is needed, or if the area used for the walk contains obstacles, the patient may fall over and clearly nursing care has become a major hazard to the patient!

PERMANENT IMMOBILITY OF GRADUAL ONSET

Intervention

Wholly compensatory

This subsystem includes the patient's internal environment as well as the external environment. The patient who is totally immobile remains a functioning human being even though one aspect of functioning may be limited. The patient should not be treated as totally unable to prevent any hazards. When living with a disabling, crippling disease, individuals get to know their bodies very well. They know how it feels when a urinary tract infection is developing or when their limbs have not been put through a range of movements or are left in an incorrect position. Thus, even though a patient may be dependent on the staff to compensate for their mobility problem, the staff in their turn must listen to what the patient is telling them and treat such information with respect. Self care means that the nurse must move away from the traditional position of thinking that she knows best.

Partially compensatory

Partially dependent patients need to work with the nursing staff to ensure that any hazard of their life, functioning or development is recognized and dealt with. Practical problems that could occur involve, for example, a mechanical fault with a wheelchair or a misunderstanding about medication after discharge. This latter point raises the issue of teaching patients self medication while they are in hospital. If patients cannot be responsible for taking medication on the ward (and the traditional drug round makes sure they are not!), should we be surprised if mistakes happen after discharge?

Educative/supportive

Patients with a long-term mobility problem often live for many years. However, it is vital that the patient receives an education programme to teach them about potential problems that may occur and become life-threatening. The role the nurse plays is essential – if a patient is discharged with no idea of, for example, the potential hazards of pressure sores, chest infections or painful, swollen calves, the nursing care has been inadequate.

Reference has already been made to self medication, and the nurse clearly has a major role in teaching patients about their drugs before discharge and subsequently in the community.

Evaluation

At the end of the day, the relevance of the individual patient's care will be seen by the presence or absence of any complications which could have been avoided. If something has gone wrong that was preventable, the nursing team must turn this into a positive event by asking why things went wrong and seeing what lessons can be learned for the future.

Promotion of normalcy

Assessment

The concept of normalcy is difficult to define. Use of the word 'normal' is inappropriate when assessing a patient since it usually refers to the nurse's view of what is normal rather than the patient's. Traditionally, psychologists have related normalcy to the individual's adjustment to the environment (Hilgard et al, 1979). They suggest that normal personality traits are those which help individuals to get on well with others and find a place in society.

Orem, in her explanation of the use of the term normalcy, lists four different aspects, which include maintaining a realistic self-concept, actively trying to develop as a human being, looking after one's own body so that it functions as well as possible, and being aware of any deviations from one's own norm and acting on that awareness.

Therefore, it is important to be able to discuss with the patient their idea of what is normal for them. Probably one of the greatest areas that has to undergo a change while in hospital is the patient's own self-image. This is more obvious when a patient is in hospital with a permanent mobility problem following trauma. However, it is also relevant when an individual has been just managing at home but has to be admitted because of a deterioration signifying that total self care will not be possible in the future. The need for nurses to be aware of a change in body image has been highlighted by writers such as Murray (1972) and Leonard (1972). Murray also explains that every stage and change in our lives is accompanied by a change in body image.

Baird (1985) has done extensive work in developing an assessment tool to help nurses diagnose altered body image in immobilized patients. She found that nurses often saw in a patient only what they wanted to see and missed cues that the patient was giving at assessment.

Goffman (1976), in his famous work on stigma, looks at the way individuals feel about being different from their perceived view of normal, and the way others or 'normals' react to those who are 'stigmatized'. He suggests that a central feature of an individual's view of being different, and therefore (in his view) suffering from a stigma, is in acceptance both from the individual and from the surrounding society. One way in which the individual is seen to cope with this is to try to rectify their handicap by surgery, medicine or quackery, and in this way they become very vulnerable to claims of instant cures. Others may cope with their 'difference' by exaggerating it and may use their helplessness to manipulate those around them to their own advantage.

Intervention

Wholly compensatory

According to Shakespeare (1975), the severity of the reaction of an individual to a total mobility problem will depend on the measure of importance placed on mobility. Thus, someone who played a lot of sport or who rated freedom of movement highly would probably have a more severe reaction than someone who hated any kind of exercise and preferred passive interests. In the studies carried out by psychologists looking at the effect of handicap, a series of recognizable reactions have been noted such as denial, anxiety, regression into the behaviour of a younger person, and an increased egocentricity when the patient becomes demanding and intolerant of the needs of others.

Shakespeare suggests that the patient's realization of the

effects of immobility is likely to occur at crisis points. These are steps and are like decision points at which the individual will have to see whether he will be able to fit into 'normal' society or have to adopt the role of the handicapped.

Patients who require this level of nursing will be constantly faced with the difference between themselves and others. Even when there are other patients with similar disabilities having to rely on nursing staff to perform even the most basic tasks for them, the individual will be constantly reminded that they are different from the vast majority of the population. Orem suggests that organizing the care of such patients so that they can establish group norms can be of help to the individual.

Partially compensatory

Helping a patient to compensate for the lack of normal mobility has practical implications for the nurse, such as encouraging a return to those leisure activities that are possible. For example, the local chess champion need not give up chess because of a mobility problem; moving the pieces may be difficult, but someone else can always be told where to move them. In addition, a whole range of sports are now available to patients in wheelchairs.

It was mentioned earlier that patients are not a static force but a dynamic one – constantly changing. Partially compensatory nursing is often caring for people who are in a transition stage, either getting better or, unfortunately, deteriorating. When patients are steadily improving and can see themselves moving to a more normal mobility state, their hopes are high, as is the motivation for practising their physiotherapy. However, for those whose condition is deteriorating and who can see their level of movement reducing, trying to find a reason why they should persevere can be difficult. It is up to the staff to be as frank as possible with the patient and not build up hopes of unrealistic goals or future plans. Individuals with a severe mobility problem are not perceived as 'normal' by any part of society around them, except perhaps within the narrow confines of a specialist unit where everybody has a mobility problem of some sort. Rather, the goals should be aimed at the slowing of the deterioration and the prevention of complications. Such patients will also need help and support in looking for new goals in their lives – other areas in which they can direct their thoughts and energies. This might be in the form of a new hobby or in taking an interest in a support group for others with similar problems. It must never be forgotten that it is the patient's prerogative to be involved or not in such pursuits and so should never be put in a position of feeling obliged to comply with the staff's wishes. Some individuals have no wish to be associated with a group of people who are not 'normal' and whom they may have disliked in the past.

Educative/supportive

For patients who are planning to return to the community, their re-education of what to expect is of paramount importance if it is not to be too traumatic an experience. Shakespeare (1975) described research which showed that non-handicapped people become much more inhibited and 'overcontrolled' in the presence of anyone with a handicap. This is due to the non-handicapped person considering each topic of conversation in case it should be tactless or hurtful to the listener. It is often thought inappropriate to talk about activites such as walking and dancing in which the relatively immobile person cannot participate. This is the sort of reaction of which the patient will have to be aware before being discharged from hospital. In fact, it is the non-handicapped person who has the problem of relating to someone with a mobility problem. If socializing with the rest of the local community is to have a chance of being successful, there needs to be an opportunity to air these problems in an open atmosphere rather than just pretending they do not exist. The person with a mobility problem will need to have time to explore the feelings that emerge about normality and what can now be considered normal for themselves compared with the past.

Before a patient is discharged into the community, weekend visits should have been arranged so that any problems can be ironed out. Even before a weekend visit can be contemplated, a visit home for an afternoon and then a full day should be tried. This not only gives the patient a chance to adjust to the very different facilities available at home, but also gives the family a chance to acclimatize to having an individual with a mobility problem in the house. Arriving home after a prolonged spell in hospital can be a very stressful time for patient and family alike. Often, a lot of organizing by many people has gone into it, and the patient is under a lot of pressure to agree that everything is wonderful. In fact, even after only a few hours in the home, the advantages of a speedy return to hospital may be uppermost in everybody's mind.

Before discharge, the family will need a comprehensive education programme in both the physical and emotional needs of the patient.

Evaluation

How well an individual overcomes any feelings of being different from the rest of society depends on many aspects of care.

The feeling of normalcy is as individual a feeling as any other. What constitutes feeling normal depends on our upbringing, our life expectations and the way we see ourself within the society in which we move. Only the patient can evaluate this aspect of care, and any help from the nursing staff to come to terms with an altered self-image, damaged self-esteem and a feeling of freakishness must be at the patient's bidding. However, for this to happen, the patient must know that there is help available and that some of the problems being faced are well documented and not in themselves out of the ordinary. To return to a psychologist's definition of normalcy, if individuals are able to adjust to their altered mobility state so that they are content with it and enjoy a level of self-esteem similar to that previously enjoyed, the care will have been successful.

DEVELOPMENTAL SELF CARE REQUISITES

Having considered self care from the point of view of the day-to-day universal requisites, we should now follow Orem's model and look at self care and development. Broadly speaking, Orem suggests that the patient needs to practise self care in two areas. First, there are the normal milestones associated with growth and maturation, and then there are more 'pathological' processes, such as social deprivation and bereavement, that interfere with normal development.

One method of incorporating these important psychosocial considerations into patient care might be to see them as added dimensions of the patient's self care that we have already discussed in the eight universal self care requisites. Thus, in planning realistic care, we need to consider the patient's development status, be they children, women of child-bearing age or the very elderly. In addition, we need to consider other negative developmental factors such as can the patient read, has he or she a permanent home or been recently bereaved? These developmental factors should therefore be included in designing a care plan around the eight universal self care requisites of Orem's model.

HEALTH DEVIATION SELF CARE REQUISITES

The individual who has a permanent mobility problem inevitably has either been ill or injured, or has some significant pathology that has resulted in an inability to move freely at will. A simple analysis of health deviancy leads to a consideration of alterations in structure, function and behaviour. We must then ask whether the patient is able to practise the required self care to deal with any problems stemming from these three areas.

Health deviation – structure

Many patients with a permanent mobility problem will have an alteration in body structure. This may be a severance of the spinal cord resulting in paraplegia, or severe joint destruction by osteoarthritis. Unfortunately, by the time the patient is recognized as having a permanent mobility problem, these deviations in structure cannot usually be altered.

What is important to nursing care is any new alteration in the structure of the patient's body. This may be the formation of a pressure sore or the presence of mouth infections due to lack of oral hygiene care by the nursing staff. A commonly seen structural change in immobile patients is dependent oedema. This can be apparent when the patient's ankles become swollen and the skin looks tight and shiny. Patients who require frequent turning may be found to have oedema of the dependent limb when lying on that side. Self care would normally consist of elevating the affected limb, but the immobile patient cannot do this. Nursing intervention is therefore required to elevate the feet on a stool with ankles as high as possible – ideally above hip level. For hand oedema, the arm should be elevated on a pillow with the hand higher than the heart.

If a generalized oedema is noted, the patient's nutritional state should be examined; a protein deficiency will lead to lack of plasma proteins and a fall in plasma protein osmotic pressure, and hence to generalized oedema. Patients should be taught what to look for and how the oedema can be reduced. Once again, we can see Orem's three nursing systems in action – compensatory, partially compensatory and educative/supportive.

Health deviation – function

Individuals who have a congenital deformity resulting in a permanent mobility problem, often do not recognize that they have a health deviation, as they have never known anything else. In the assessment, the nurse will be looking for an alteration in the functional levels of the patient. What can they not do now that they could three months ago? What help do they require now in their day-to-day living that they did not need three months ago? Changes in function do not usually occur overnight and, in patients with a permanent mobility problem, it is essential that the nurse has some means of regular assessment so that changes can be measured rather than allowed to occur gradually, almost unnoticed. When there is a relatively sharp reduction in level of self care, the patient should be assessed for an acute problem overriding the long-term one, such as an acute infection, which is making them feel unwell.

Health deviation – behaviour

The behavioural response to a permanent mobility problem has been discussed already. One area that has not been examined, however, is the patient questioning why it happened to them. This type of question inevitably must be one of the first to be asked following sudden onset immobility and will be dealt with in the following chapter. However, it is a question that will also be raised from time to time, often by older immobile patients in a reflective mood when they are looking at their lives and thinking how different it would have been without arthritis or polio or the congenital deformity that has wrecked at least this one aspect of their lives. This self questioning may be followed by a time of depression and moodiness, and the patient and staff should be aware of this. It is unreasonable to expect anyone to go through life without periods when a dark cloud appears to hang over them. This must be especially so for those who are unable to fulfill the twentieth century's ideal of a mobile, independent, youthful individual.

In her deeper explanation of health deviation, Orem looks not only at abnormal self care requisites due to disease and altered pathological states, but also at those due to medical interventions and investigations. The relevance this has to patients with a permanent mobility problem lies in their acceptance of medical intervention and their understanding of why it is necessary at this stage. The need to wear an orthotic appliance requires a certain amount of patient compliance if it is to be of any use, and yet such an appliance may seriously affect a patient's self care ability. Patients must also be aware of any dangers associated with the medical treatment they are receiving, such as the use of steroids for severe rheumatoid arthritis or the chances of joint replacements becoming loose within 2–3 years and requiring further surgery. The whole subject of informed consent needs far more publicity among patients who are quite willing to accept that the method of treatment offered by their doctor is the only one of choice. Orem suggests that, if self care is the goal of patients, then they are the individuals who will have to live with the consequences of the prescribed treatment.

References

Abramson L., Seligman M., Teasedale J. (1978). Learned helplessness in humans; critique and reformulation. *Journal of Abnormal Psychology*, 87, (1), 49–74.

Baird S. (1985). Development of a nursing assessment tool to diagnose altered body image in immobilised patients. *Orthopaedic Nursing*, 4, 47–53.

Ben-Schlomo L., Short M. (1985). The effects of physical conditioning on selected dimensions of self-concept in sedentary females. *Occupational Therapy in Mental Health*, 5 (4), 27–43.

Burford K., Pentland B. (1985). Management of motor neuron disease: the physiotherapist's role. *Physiotherapy*, 71(9), 402–404.

Downie P., ed. (1984). *Cash's Textbook of Orthopaedics and Rheumatology for Physiotherapists*. London: Faber and Faber.

Egerton J. (1986). Nursing the patient with a spinal cord injury. In *A.B.C. of Spinal Cord Injury*. London: British Medical Journal.

Goffman E. (1976). *Stigma*. Baltimore: Penguin.

Goldberg W., Fitzpatrick J. (1980). Movement therapy with the aged. *Nursing Research*, 29 (6), 339–346.

Hickey J. (1986). *Neurological and Neurosurgical Nursing*. Philadelphia: Lippincott.

Hilgard E., Atkinson R., Atkinson R. (1979). *Introduction to Psychology*. New York: Harcourt Brace Jovanovich, Inc.

Leonard B.J. (1972). Body image changes in chronic illness. *Nursing Clinics of North America*, 7 (4), 687–695.

Murray R.L. (1972). Body image development in adulthood. *Nursing Clinics of North America*, 7 (4), 696–707.

Moody M. (1989). *Incontinence*. London: Heinemann. In press.

Orem D. (1985). *Nursing: Concepts of Practice*. New York: McGraw-Hill.

Shakespeare R. (1975). *The Psychology of Handicap*. London: Methuen.

Bibliography

Burke D., Murray D. (1975). *Handbook of Spinal Cord Medicine*. London: Macmillan.

McCann V.J. (1979). The prevention of depression in the immobilised patient. *Orthopaedic Nursing*, 6, 433–438.

Schoen D.C. (1986). *The Nursing Process in Orthopaedics*. Connecticut: Appleton-Century-Crofts.

Walsh M. (1985). *Accident and Emergency Nursing: A New Approach*. London: Heinemann.

6

The patient with permanent immobility of sudden onset

The effect of sudden onset immobility on both the individual and the family can never be underestimated. In the instant it takes for a cerebral artery to rupture or for a person to fall down some steps, the chairman of a multinational corporation or an international football star may lose their ability to move at will and become dependent on others forever. Whatever the cause of the immobility, there will have been no preparations made, no time to become accustomed to the idea, no time to make alterations to a lifestyle.

In this chapter, the immediate care of individuals who have suddenly become immobile will be examined in detail. Three principal causes of such sudden and permanent immobility will be considered; trauma, viral infections of the spinal cord and a cerebrovascular accident. The central theme will be the relationship between the patient's medical condition and nursing care, looking at both from the patient's inability to move at will. This means that the more general aspects of care will be omitted from this chapter as they can be found in other parts of the book to which the reader will be directed when appropriate.

If traumatic causes of sudden permanent immobility are split into three major subgroups, we have the following five groups of patients to consider:
1. Spinal cord injury.
2. Traumatic amputation of one or both lower limbs.
3. Severe head injury.

4. Acute anterior poliomyelitis.
5. Cerebrovascular accident.

SPINAL CORD INJURY

The prognosis for patients suffering a spinal cord injury has improved dramatically since the early part of the century. In the first world war, 90% of patients with a spinal cord injury died within one year and only 1% survived for 20 years (Swain et al, 1986). However, even in the 1960s, the mortality rate associated with quadriplegia remained high at 35%. As a result, Regional Spinal Cord Injuries Units were set up, where staff with specialist expertise could care for such patients. Unfortunately, an injury sustained at the time of an accident may be compounded by the inappropriate action of those rendering first aid. An even sadder situation occurs when the original injury is made worse by staff at the receiving hospital who should know better but who fail to make an accurate assessment of the patient. Frequently, the poor general condition of the patient makes transfer to a specialist unit impossible for several days. During this time, other complications may set in simply because the staff are unused to such injuries and are worried about making the situation worse. They therefore fail to move the patient adequately so that pressure sores develop, or fail to ensure that the bladder wall is never overstretched, thus delaying the return of bladder function; these would seem to be the two major complications for which general hospitals are blamed by the specialist units.

A large proportion of spinal cord injuries occur in the cervical area (55%, as opposed to 35% in the thoracic region and 10% in the lumbar region) and are the result of road traffic accidents. In road accidents, motor cyclists fare worse, with an incidence twice that of car drivers.

Although spinal cord injury is usually associated with fracture of a vertebra, the two do not necessarily go together. Stability of the spine is maintained, not only by the shape of the vertebrae but by a highly efficient system of ligaments (see Fig. 6.1). Although X-rays obviously have an important part to play in the assessment of any possible spinal cord damage, they do not show the ligamentous damage nor the amount of

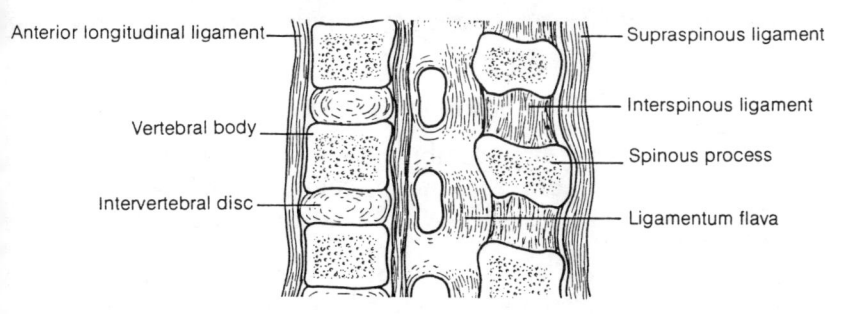

Anterior longitudinal ligament
Vertebral body
Intervertebral disc
Supraspinous ligament
Interspinous ligament
Spinous process
Ligamentum flava

Fig. 6.1 *The spinal ligaments*

disruption that might have occurred at the time of the accident.

The main aim of all care, once the patient is admitted to hospital, is maintenance of alignment of the vertebral column, protection of the cord from any more damage and prevention of any further complications. Complete severance of the spinal cord does not always occur. The effect of the injury will depend on which fibres of the cord have been damaged beyond repair and which have been simply bruised but will eventually function again.

Complete transection

Most injuries to the spinal cord result in damage to the upper motor neuron. This is shown by a total loss of voluntary movement below the lesion but with the presence of spinal reflexes. As spinal reflexes are dependent on central control to 'damp them down', loss of this influence results in spasticity.

When the lesion is below L1, the damage occurs to the cauda equina, a collection of lower motor neurons, as the spinal cord ends at T12. This results in total flaccid paralysis, loss of spinal reflexes and muscle wasting.

When there is complete severance of the spinal cord, the sensory pathways carrying pain, touch, heat and cold are also lost below the lesion. Following these very severe injuries, not only are the motor and sensory functions altered but the autonomic nerve fibres are also interrupted, leading to problems of hypotension due to loss of vasomotor control.

Loss of control over temperature and bowel and bladder function also occur.

Incomplete lesions

In these injuries, any combination of effects may occur. However, there are recognized combinations which are classed as syndromes. Of these the most important are:

1. Acute anterior cervical spinal cord syndrome. There is usually complete loss of motor function below the lesion, loss of pain, temperature and touch but preservation of proprioception, light touch and position (that is, the posterior columns remain intact).
2. Brown-Séquard Syndrome. This occurs when there is damage to one side of the spinal cord, as occurs in lateral hyperextension injuries. The lesion will be manifested by decreased or increased pain, temperature, and touch sensation on one side along with complete motor paralysis below the lesion. On the opposite side, there will be loss of pain, touch and temperature sensation as those tracts cross soon after entering the cord. From a functional point of view, usually the limb with the poorest sensation has the best motor function and vice versa.
3. Cauda equina lesions. Because of the mobility of the cauda equina, these lesions are often incomplete and the neurological damage unpredictable. The nerve roots may be damaged either on one side or both, but as long as they are not actually severed they do have the ability to regenerate.

Spinal shock is a phenomenon that occurs after severe spinal cord injury in which there is a marked flaccidity below the level of the lesion. At first, this may be accompanied by reflex activity, although eventually this too disappears. The spinal shock may last from a few hours to several weeks, but the speed or extent of the return of nerve activity can never be predicted.

Maintenance of alignment of the vertebral column

Patients with an injury to the cervical vertebrae are usually first nursed in some form of skeletal traction. This allows the patient to be moved, albeit with great care, and helps in the reduction of fractures. Following a dislocation of the vertebrae, one of the major methods of reducing the fracture is gentle distraction (1–2 kg) with skull traction. Unlike dislocations of other joints the short, sharp pull of a manipulation to re-oppose the articular surfaces is inappropriate in this instance! Skull traction may be applied using a pair of tongs or calipers which are inserted into either side of the skull (see Fig. 6.2) or a halo brace (see Fig. 6.3).

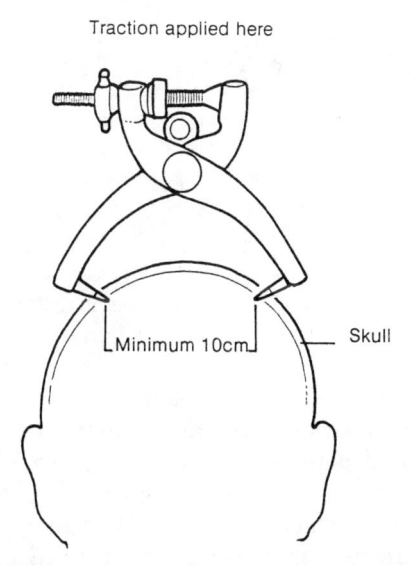

Fig. 6.2 *Crutchfield calipers used to apply skeletal traction to the skull in the treatment of fractures of cervical vertebrae*

While on skull traction, patients are usually nursed on either a Stryker turning frame or a Stoke Egerton bed (see pages 90 and 91). Whenever either of these beds is used, it is extremely important that the staff are competent in their use and that, during patient turning, there is a nominated person who will ensure that the patient's neck remains in alignment with the rest of the body. In some units, the importance of the nurse holding the head during turns is recognized by making it an extended nursing role. The pin sites of the calipers or tongs should be treated in the same way as the pin sites of any other type of skeletal traction; that is, they should be checked daily

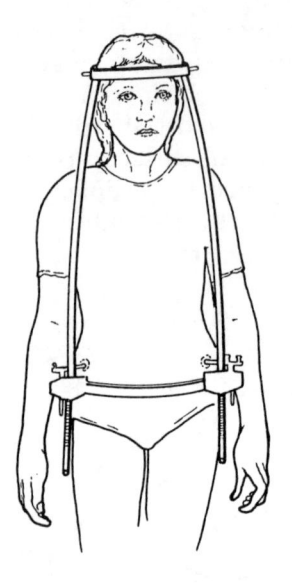

Fig. 6.3 *An example of a halo brace, often referred to as halopelvic traction*

for any signs of infection and kept clean with the use of an antiseptic cream when necessary. The position of the calipers should be noted as they do occasionally jump out of position. This could prove very distressing to the patient as well as harmful. Skeletal traction usually lasts for 6–8 weeks, after which the patient has a soft collar applied and is gradually introduced to the sitting position. This may be done very efficiently by using the profiling bed (see page 99) and the patient must be carefully monitored for postural hypotension.

The use of halo braces is increasing. They have the obvious advantage of allowing the patient to sit up and, when there is minimal spinal cord damage, to commence mobilizing. When caring for a patient in such a brace, the nurse must again check the pin sites for any signs of infection and that the position of the brace is unchanged. The nuts which hold the supports to the halo itself must be checked daily as these can slowly loosen.

Patients who have suffered a spinal cord injury in the lower spine will be nursed free in bed but require turning every two hours with a team of at least five people. The most important person in this team is the one holding the head and ensuring that the spine remains in a straight line. To do this, the 'head nurse' stands behind the patient's head and checks that the nose is in line with the sternum which is in line with the symphysis pubis. Once the alignment is confirmed, the patient's neck is gently supported by the nurse's hands and the head supported by the forearms.

During lifting with a five-person team, three stand to one side of the patient; the right arm of the nurse nearest the patient's head is inserted under the shoulders and the left arm under the waist, the middle nurse inserts the right arm under the waist and the left arm under the patient's hips, and the third nurse inserts the right arm under the patient's thighs and the left arm under the ankles. Although this appears a complicated system, it is all done in sequence and each time an arm is inserted under the patient the fourth member of the team applies counter pressure from the opposite side to prevent any spinal movement. The fifth person throughout is responsible for the head and neck alignment. Once the lift is completed, the arms of the lifters are removed from under the patient in reverse order, again with the fourth member of the team applying counter traction to prevent spinal movement. At all times, the natural shape of the spine, that is the maintenance of all curves, should be retained by the use of neck rolls and supportive pillows.

Prevention of further complications

The prevention of pressure sores is one of the major demands on nurses when caring for patients immediately following a spinal cord injury. Neglect in these early days can mean months of dressings and intensive nursing care to promote healing. Patients with diminished sensation in the skin will be prone to sores, and of course, if they do feel sore, they cannot change their position. In fact, they are positively discouraged from making any movement, thus compounding the problem. Good preventative care in these early days is essential.

Paralytic ileus usually accompanies spinal cord injuries and often lasts about a week. Burke and Murray (1975) suggest that unrecognized paralytic ileus is the commonest underlying cause of sudden death in the quadriplegic patient in the first 48 hours since it may cause the patient to inhale vomit. Another complication of paralytic ileus may be dehydration. To prevent these complications of paralytic ileus, the patient with a spinal cord injury should not be given anything orally, should have a nasogastric tube inserted which should be aspirated, and an intravenous infusion should be commenced. The return of bowel sounds and passing of flatus should signify the end of the paralytic ileus period.

Paralysis of the intercostal muscles will occur following a spinal cord injury above the level of C7, and paralysis of the diaphragm will occur in a lesion above the level of C4. When the patient retains the use of the diaphragm but not the intercostal muscles for breathing, it will take a little while for the body to adjust to this altered state. Signs of hypoxia should be looked for and, if necessary, the patient should be ventilated. A tidal volume of 200 cc or a vital capacity of 800 cc are thought to be sufficient for basic requirements for a quadriplegic patient. A blood gas estimation of Po_2 60 mmHg is thought adequate, as is a Pco_2 of 45–50 mmHg for a quadriplegic patient.

The neurogenic bladder is one which has been compromised by the alteration of the nerve supply. In the first few days following a spinal cord injury, the patient should be catheterized to prevent retention and urinary overflow. An upper motor lesion will result in the return of the spinal arc emptying reflex once spinal shock has passed, although the patient will not experience any feeling of fullness and therefore be unaware that he is about to void urine. The capacity of the bladder may be less than usual. In a patient with a lower motor neuron lesion, the function of the bladder will be governed by stretch reflexes. In this instance, the incontinence experienced by the patient will be overflow and the bladder will not empty properly.

Once spinal shock has resolved, the patient can be assessed for the suitability of a bladder training programme. The main aim is to test for the adequacy of the perineal nerve supply and detrusor autonomic supply. Investigations which may be performed include a cystometrogram, voiding cystogram and an intravenous pyelogram. The aim of all bladder management is that the patient should eventually be catheter-free. In patients with an upper motor neuron lesion, emptying the bladder by stimulating reflex contraction can be initiated by finding the 'trigger point'.

In patients with a lower motor neurone lesion, although the bladder is denervated, the detrusor mechanism has some inbuilt contractile ability which can be used as long as the bladder has not been overstretched in the past. This underlines the importance of correct bladder management in the first few days before transfer to a specialist unit. External pressure will be required to empty such a bladder, either by increasing intra-abdominal pressure or by manual pressure.

The spasticity which results from an upper motor neuron lesion usually occurs within 6–10 weeks after injury. The two main patterns of spasticity are flexor and extensor, neither of which can be attributed to either complete or incomplete lesions. As an extensor is of more functional use than a flexor spasticity, the joints should be put through a range of movement to tire the stretch reflex which causes the flexion. The limbs should always be positioned in such a way that flexion is reduced. Hydrotherapy may be used to overcome flexor spasticity, as may the application of heated pads to joints. Occasionally, drugs such as diazepam may be used to reduce spasticity. The main complication of flexor spasticity is shortening of muscle tendons and joint contractures. Again, the care given in the first few days has a bearing on the overall recovery of the patient.

One of the drawbacks of the development of spinal units is that the staff of general hospitals have little experience in the care of spinally injured patients. Those who do have a chance to care for such patients immediately after injury have no opportunity to evaluate the care they give in the early stages in the light of the patient's ultimate lifestyle. This would suggest the advisability of staff from trauma units in busy general hospitals attending study days in spinal units so that they can see the whole concept of care over 9–12 months rather than just 2–7 days.

TRAUMATIC AMPUTATIONS OF ONE OR BOTH LOWER LIMBS

The injuries included in this part of the chapter are surgical amputations carried out at the scene of an accident to facilitate freeing the victim from wreckage, amputations that occur due to the violence of the accident itself and amputations that take place subsequently in hospital after a fight to save the limb.

Whatever the reason for the amputation, the end result is much the same and the goals of treatment remain saving as much of the limb as possible, preventing complications and helping the patient to adapt, both physically and emotionally, to the inevitable reduction in mobility.

Following traumatic amputation of a limb at an accident, the immediate care will be concentrated on saving life which will be threatened by haemorrhage and wound contamination (gas gangrene and tetanus). If the amputation is due to a crushing injury, there will be a larger amount of tissue damage above the level of the amputation than if the injury was due to a 'clean severance'. The patient will require surgery immediately to remove any tissue that is dead or of dubious viability, together with contaminating material, and for ligation of blood vessels; assessment of the viability of the stump is also required.

The level of the amputation is crucial to the mobility that can be expected afterwards. Following a below-knee amputation, the individual who was fairly fit and active before the accident could expect to resume most, if not all, of the activities. Even squash and running have been successfully continued with a below-knee prosthesis. An above-knee amputation will have a much greater effect on the mobility of the individual as the knee joint, so essential to mobility, is difficult to replace artificially. The energy requirements to walk with an above-knee prosthesis are also much higher than those required in normal walking. For the older patient, this level of energy requirement may make walking any further than around the house prohibitive.

The two main types of amputation are the flap type and the guillotine type. The former is used when there is not thought to be any contamination present and the wound has a good chance of healing. The anterior flap is usually longer than the posterior flap so that the suture line can be well to the back of the stump. This facilitates weight bearing on the stump at a later date. The guillotine type of amputation is used when it is considered that the wound might become infected. The skin and soft tissues are severed at the same level as the bone and the wound is left open to drain. It may be closed at a later date when any infection has been dealt with and any necrotic tissue removed.

The specific postoperative care of the patient following an amputation lies in ensuring optimum conditions for wound healing to take place, the prevention of complications such as joint contractures, and helping the patient to adapt to the effect of suddenly discovering the loss of a limb. This latter effect will lead to the patient having to work through the grieving process to come to terms with their loss.

Following an amputation, the stump is usually encased in a crepe bandage applied in such a way that the distal part of the stump is under the greatest pressure (see Fig. 6.4). Traditionally, this bandage was reapplied at least daily, the rationale being that it would improve the shape of the stump and make it more suitable to fit into a prosthesis. This theory has now fallen into disrepute mainly, it has to be said, because the standards of stump bandaging performed by most nurses was so bad. The effect was that pressure was greatest around the proximal end of the limb, forcing fluid into the distal end and thus making the end of the stump bulbous.

Occasionally, a pillow may be placed under the stump to aid drainage and reduce oedema. However, this should be used only in extreme cases as the effect on the hip is to encourage a flexion deformity – a recognized complication of above-knee amputations in any case as patients spend a large proportion of their time during the recovery stages sitting with the hip in flexion. The shortness of the above-knee stump and the action of the strong hip flexor muscles (iliacus and psoas muscles) combine to increase the likelihood of a hip flexion deformity. To overcome this, the patient should lie prone at least twice a day – care being taken that the hip is in full extension and also the breathing is not compromised in any way. Many patients find lying on their stomachs most uncomfortable and try very hard to avoid it. One of the nurse's prime responsibilities is to ensure that the patient knows exactly why this exercise has to be carried out in order to gain their full cooperation.

In a below-knee amputation, the patient is in danger of developing a knee flexion deformity and, as soon as possible

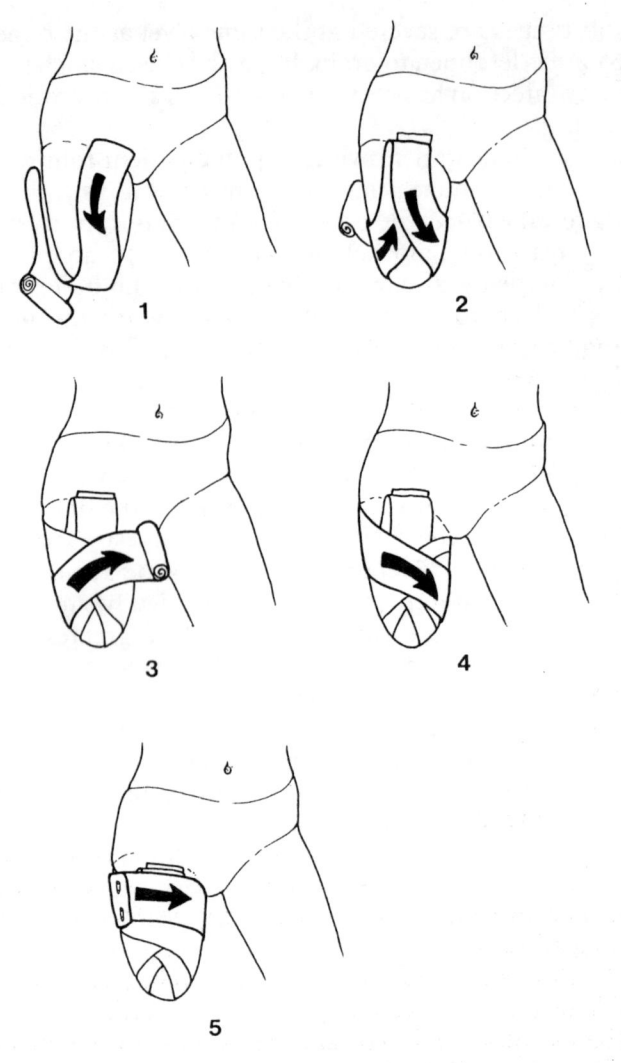

Fig. 6.4 *Traditional bandaging method of an above-knee stump*

after surgery, knee extension exercises should be encouraged to avoid shortening of the hamstring muscles.

Once the patient has recovered from the anaesthetic, both the nurse and the physiotherapist will be encouraging mobility with either a frame or crutches. In the case of a bilateral amputee, a wheelchair should be provided so that the patient retains a feeling of mobility. Once the stitches are removed from the wound, a PAM aid may be used. This is a multi-fit pylon which is inflated around the stump and gives the patient with an above-knee amputation a feeling of walking while taking the weight through the ischial tuberosity.

Unlike patients who have an amputation for peripheral vascular disease, patients with a traumatic amputation will have been unable to discuss the effects of the operation on themselves and the rest of their family. Awakening from a major operation to be told that a leg or even both legs have been amputated will be catastrophic, especially when the limb(s) can still be felt. Time will be needed for the patient to work through the grieving process to come to terms with the feeling of loss.

Kelly (1985) has linked the grieving which occurs following major surgery to that experienced following death. The grieving model he looked at was that described by Parkes (1972) and he considers it from his own personal experiences. Parkes identified four stages of grieving:
1. Realization
2. A time of alarm
3. A time of searching
4. A feeling of internal loss and mutilation.

Kelly describes these stages as a continuum, one stage running into another. At first, he felt a certain reality shock as he realized that the surgery actually had been performed and this took several days to become apparent as the full effects of the general anaesthetic wore off. A stage of denial, when the patient will not want to accept what has happened, may precede this time. The realization was quite quickly followed by a time of alarm when Kelly became totally pre-occupied with the hospital surroundings and showed a lack of interest with life outside. During the stage of searching, which could correspond to a time of extreme depression and rejection, Kelly was continually asking 'why?'. The final stage was associated with a time of anger and hatred against the staff while feeling mutilated and stigmatized.

Kelly suggests that, because the post-surgical state is an altered state, the individual will never be sure what his or her reactions to it will be, or for that matter what the reactions of others will be. For many, their background knowledge will not include how to cope with his new situation. Parkes suggests that the newly bereaved person feels in much the same way.

Towards the end of his essay, Kelly suggests that the significance of the knowledge of this grieving process in patients, following major surgery when they have lost a part of their body, lies in the way nurses are taught to care for such individuals. If the nursing care is aimed only at physical care, the patient will not have the opportunity to recover emotionally. Unfortunately, it is physical care that nurses feel most at home with while emotional care is frequently overlooked by staff. It is also suggested that a busy surgical or trauma ward is not the ideal place for discussion of the grieving process with the patient. A final point was that nurses often perceive a patient's grief reaction as self-pity or manipulative behaviour which is not to be encouraged.

Tagliacozzo and Mauksch (1972) suggest that a physical illness allows the patient to become dependent on others for their basic care for a while, whereas to become emotionally dependent is acceptable only in a very few instances. If the patient is to benefit from planned individualized care, the emotional care must be of as high a standard as the physical care.

Phantom limb

This phenomenon following an amputation includes itching, tingling and burning, as well as pain. It is estimated that 5–10% of patients experience some degree of phantom limb pain. Usually, this type of pain occurs immediately after the operation, but for some people it intensifies over the weeks following surgery. There is not necessarily any relationship between the amount of stump pain and phantom limb pain that the individual suffers. Following traumatic amputations, patients have been found less likely to suffer phantom limb pains than were those who had had severe pain in their leg preoperatively. For patients who do suffer this postoperative complication, several factors may trigger it, such as touching the stump, emotional stress and fatigue. The pathophysiology is not completely understood and therefore its treatment is highly subjective. Some patients find non-addictive analgesia sufficient, whereas for some patients even transection of the sensory pathways does not completely relieve it.

SEVERE HEAD INJURY

Damage to the brain following a head injury may be mild and reversible or severe and irreversible. In the most severe brain injuries, the victim does not survive; however, some individuals do survive serious injuries only to be left with a large motor deficit.

The immediate nursing care of a patient with a severe head injury is obviously aimed at survival, and so the maintenance of an adequate airway, breathing and circulation (the ABC of resuscitation) and careful monitoring for any deterioration and development of complications, is of prime importance.

As the brain is closely confined within the skull, there is little room for any swelling. Therefore, the development of cerebral oedema must be kept to a minimum if brain compression and damage is to be avoided. To help to achieve this, the blood CO_2 levels should be kept low using high concentrations of oxygen, usually via a Hudson mask. The use of intravenous fluids should also be carefully watched to prevent over infusion and generalized fluid overload.

The level of consciousness should be monitored from the time of the accident, at very frequent intervals as this is the most sensitive indication of developing complications. An objective system of recording consciousness levels should be used, such as the Glasgow Coma Scale, which will include the level of motor function in the patient's upper and lower limbs. Walsh (1985) suggests the importance of the same nurse performing the observations to avoid the risk of changes which might be recorded being due to different personnel rather than to real changes in the patient. The same nurse doing the observations is more likely to detect changes than is a succession of different nurses. An initial observation frequency might be as often as five minutes, although 15 minutes is more common, proceeding to half-hourly as the patient appears more stable.

Following a severe head injury with a long recovery time, the development of contractures causes great difficulties for the nurse and physiotherapist when trying to mobilize the patient. The use of a tilt table in the very early stages of treatment to allow weight-bearing, reduce contractures of hips and knees and to help dorsiflexion of the ankle. If this is done, care should be taken to ensure that the patient's heels are in touch with the floor.

If more severe contractures occur, serial plaster cylinders may be used. Plasters are applied around the joint and, after a few days, a wedge is inserted opening out the joint and stretching the muscles. When the plasters are removed 10–14 days later, the contracture is usually reduced. Another plaster is then applied and the whole process repeated. Joints which are suitable for treatment in this way are the knees, ankles and elbows.

If serial plasters are unsuccessful in the treatment of contractures, surgery may be contemplated. However, these operations are not without their complications and, at the end of the day, the patient might be worse off than with the contracture.

The effect of head injuries on mobility will depend on which part of the brain is affected by the injury. The motor cortex which controls voluntary movement is located anterior to the central sulcus (see page 10). Any damage to this area will result in a reduction of the individual's ability to move at will. The type of disordered motor function will vary greatly and include spasticity, rigidity and loss of coordination. There are often proprioception problems and sensory disorders which will affect motor function.

Very often, the whole unit of motor function will be affected and so the musculature will be uneven. Bobath (1980) has suggested that muscles which appear weak are often only weak in comparison with the strength of the opposing spastic muscle groups. It would appear that spasticity is the greatest physical problem of the head injured patient.

Much like children develop their motor function in various steps, following a severe head injury the patient will need to move through various well-established stages. The first and most important one is to learn head control followed by eye focus. This should be followed by stability of the shoulder girdle to allow hands and arms to be brought into the midline. Only when this proximal stability has been established can the patient learn any kind of controlled hand activity. The next stage to be mastered is balance when standing, and only then can the patient be taught to walk again.

In the majority of patients, control comes proximally before distally, and that the degree of that control can be influenced by the position of the head and body. Patients with a large sensory loss make a poorer recovery than those with less sensory loss. However, the degree of sensory loss can be difficult to assess as the patient will often not be able to concentrate for any length of time.

As spasticity is one of the major complications which slows down recovery, much of the nurse's and the physiotherapist's time is spent trying to overcome it. A fairly recent innovation in the care of patients following head injury is the use of a very large inflatable ball and an inflated mattress. The mattress provides an environment which is supportive but in which the patient's weight is evenly distributed, not just at the boney prominences but over a much greater body area. This reduces sensory stimulation and also reflex activity. By rolling the patient around the mattress the muscle spasm is seen to be reduced. The beach ball is used to lay the patient over so that the feeling of movement is not lost. By gently rolling the ball the patient can learn to keep the neck extended and to gain some control of the head, which will reduce muscle spasm. While exercising with the beach ball, the patient can begin to learn postural adjustment, which again will help in the reduction of spasticity. Once some head and neck control has been learned and there is some reduction in muscle spasm, the patient can be sat on the ball and gently rocked to allow changes in position to be experienced.

In the early days of rehabilitation following severe head injury, the use of a tilt table can be of great help, especially in those with severe flexor spasticity. It allows the patient to retain some feeling of weight-bearing, and care should be taken that weight is taken through the calcaneums. Once the patient has some control of movement, the use of the tilt table should be phased out.

Dyspraxia refers to the patient's inability to sequence the gait correctly. The aim of treatment is to tackle one sequence of movement at a time and only then to move on to another one. This will involve the constant repetition of the one movement so that eventually the patient can reproduce it spontaneously. When the patient can interrupt the sequence of movement or alter its speed, the treatment will be considered to have been successful. Some patients will be unable to visualize the required pattern of movement and, in this situation, the nurse and physiotherapist will have to give repeated demonstrations. The use of a video might also be of benefit.

Even when the patient is thought to have mastered one particular sequence of movement, constant reinforcement will be required to ensure that the progress is not short-lived and to avoid regression.

A further obstacle to mobility may be cerebellar incoordination in which the patient has as full range of movement but no control over it. The general aims of treatment with such patients are mobility with stability. This is achieved by emphasis on patterns of movement rather than static exercises, and the use of weighted aids has been found to be of great benefit in helping to control the lack of coordination. These aids include weighted waistcoats to help patients who are ataxic, and weighted caps to help patients with poor head control. These weighted aids, however, should be used for only a short time as there is evidence to suggest that patients adjust to their effect, thus invalidating any benefit.

The effect of a severe head injury on an individual's mobility can be devastating in its severity and permanence. An optimistic approach is required not only for the patient but also for the family, for whom the period in hospital may be just the beginning of a very long rehabilitation period in which they play a large part. Various support groups have developed for the families of such patients and these can be of great practical help with useful suggestions which may make life a little easier. They may also provide a much needed understanding shoulder to cry on, as well as unexpected assistance such as car transport to visit the hospital or physiotherapy department, some cash to help pay for a short holiday for the family, or someone to care for the victim while the rest of the family have a break.

ACUTE ANTERIOR POLIOMYELITIS (INFANTILE PARALYSIS)

The incidence of this infectious disease which can affect the nervous system has, on the whole, been eradicated in the Western world due to the widespread use of the Sabin vaccine in baby immunization programmes. However, outbreaks do occur, especially as the public are lulled into a false sense of security. The causative virus is found in the nose of infected individuals and the mouth is thought to be the means of entry to the body. The summer and autumn are times when it is most prevalent and it tends to affect young adults and children.

The infected person needs to be isolated for 10–14 days during which time symptoms of a 'flu-like' illness will manifest themselves, along with signs of nervous irritation such as altered reflexes and an increased number of white blood cells in the cerebrospinal fluid. For some, this will be the extent of the illness. For others, it will progress to the more severe form of the disease and affect the anterior horn cell of the spinal cord (spinal paralytic poliomyelitis). Besides a paralysis, which will vary according to the level of the cord affected, the patient will experience pain and tenderness in the affected muscles. The paralysis will be flaccid, as it is a condition of the lower motor neuron, with loss of reflexes leading to muscle wasting and underdevelopment of limbs.

During the early paralytic phase, the patient may need sedation and analgesia to reduce pain and restlessness, as these factors are thought to increase the extent of the paralysis. The limbs should be handled very carefully during any change of position to ensure that no overstretching of the joints occurs. Once this early stage has passed, the affected limbs will need to be put through a range of passive movements on a regular basis. Various splints may be used to support a drop foot or dropped wrist, and joints should be observed for contractures. As the severity of the disease lessens, there should be a gradual improvement in the patient's condition, although for those with permanent damage to the motor neuron, paralysis of the muscle it supplies will be permanent. While the disease is still active, the patient should be carefully observed for involvement of the respiratory muscles, especially if the arm muscles appear to be weak – indicating involvement in the cervical area.

In the long term, orthoses such as a toe spring may be required to overcome such disabilities as foot drop (see Fig. 6.5), or surgery may be performed to transplant tendons of

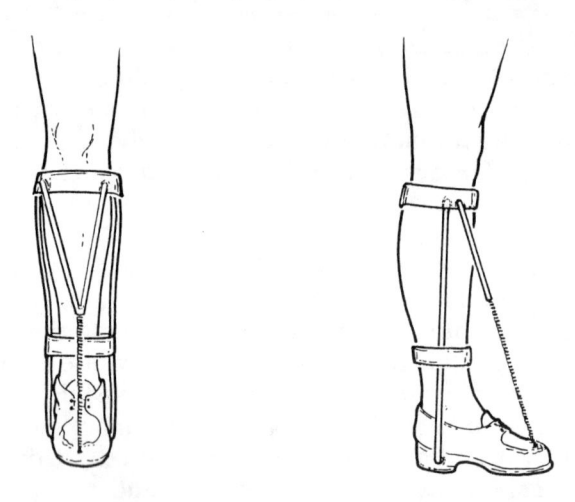

Fig. 6.5 *Toe-sprung orthosis used to overcome foot drop*

functioning muscles to areas of non-functioning muscles to provide the patient with a better functional limb. Arthrodesis of joints may help to overcome joint deformity due to paralysis of some muscle groups. Long-term physiotherapy will also be required to re-educate some muscles to overcome the paralysis of others.

CEREBROVASCULAR ACCIDENT (CVA)

The pathology of cerebrovascular accidents has been discussed in Chapter One. Although there are many reasons why CVA may occur, the effect is the same – the death of an area of brain tissue. Following a cerebral haemorrhage, there may be an increase in intracranial pressure, as the blood cannot readily escape the closed vault of the skull. This may potentially add to the damage caused to the brain tissue. When the part affected is the motor area, the patient will experience a loss of voluntary motor function on the opposite side of the body (see Fig. 1.2). As this is a condition of the upper motor neuron, the patient will suffer a spastic paralysis as the spinal reflexes will continue to function in an exaggerated manner.

Occasionally, the patient may experience a 'warning' in the form of a transient loss of motor or sensory function or a feeling of light headedness before the stroke. Patients known to have predisposing factors to cerebrovascular accidents, such as hypertension or atherosclerosis, should be made aware of these warning signals.

In the early days following a stroke, the nursing care will be aimed at helping to preserve the patient's life by intensive support of the various physiological systems (airway, hydration etc.) and avoiding the familiar complications of immobility that we have discussed so far. Once this stage has passed, however, the patient will need help to overcome the motor deficit and commence mobilizing.

One of the most common effects of a stroke is hemiplegia, and in the first few days this is usually shown by a marked loss of muscle tone and flaccidity. It is only after a few days that the spinal reflex action returns and the limbs on the affected side become spastic. There may also be a sensory loss on the same side as the motor deficit. The typical paralysis of a stroke hemiplegic patient is that of an individual whose forearm is adducted and elbow, wrist, fingers and thumb are flexed. In the lower limb, the hip is externally rotated and there is flexion of the hip and knee with plantar flexion of the ankle. If the joints are left like this, the joint capsule, ligaments and tendons become dense and firm and permanently contracted and shortened. Consequently, from the onset of the CVA it is essential that the patient's joints are put through a range of passive movements, so that the structures around the joints are stretched and prevented from shortening.

To encourage good limb position, the affected arm should be placed on a pillow at 90° to the trunk with a roll of bandage or foam in the hand in a functional position. Sometimes, a splint may be required to prevent contracture of the fingers. To reduce the effects of external rotation of the hip, a firm pillow or sandbag should be placed along the length of the patient's leg. The use of a footboard or splint should keep the ankle at right angles. Due to the strength of the flexors of the knee and hip, the patient should lie prone at least twice a day for 30 minutes each time to prevent contracture.

Once the patient's general condition has improved sufficiently, an assessment of the help required to commence mobilizing must be made. Once weight-bearing on the affected side begins, patients react in one of two ways. Either the weight-bearing produces an extensor spasm of the limb or a flexor spasm. It is fortunate that most patients experience an extensor spasm, which stabilizes the affected leg while the unaffected leg is carrying through in the gait sequence. If the patient experiences a flexor spasm, the affected leg will not weight-bear and the patient will require an orthosis, such as a caliper or brace, to support the bodyweight.

Some patients will suffer a loss of proprioception (knowledge of joint position in space) which will make their gait ataxic and awkward. For most patients, their rehabilitation towards self care will be aimed at making themselves as independent as possible, and this will often need to be taught. Some exercises will be required to strengthen the muscles that will have to take over from those affected, and the patient should be taught these exercises and given the responsibility of carrying them out the recommended number of times per day.

The expertise of the occupational therapist will help the patient to obtain any gadgets which might make self care a little easier. These may include rims to fit on plates against which the food can be pushed to help to get it onto a spoon, or handles to fit on cutlery to aid gripping.

Following a CVA, the rehabilitative process is long and arduous for both the patient and the family. This is not helped by the patient's labile emotional state and communication difficulty if, for example, the speech centre in the brain is also affected.

Sometimes, there is also an impairment of intellectual skills which particularly adds to the family's distress. This distress may be eased by joining a support group for the families and victims of cerebrovascular accidents.

SUMMARY

If the sort of situations considered in this chapter have a common theme running through them, it is the suddenness with which the patient finds mobility severely and permanently impaired. More than ever, the patient is going to think 'why me?'

This underlines the importance of the nurse thinking beyond physical care to the psychological and sociological dimensions of what is involved. As we saw in the last chapter, the use of Orem's model of nursing should facilitate such an approach, as well as being most appropriate to the self care situation in which these patients will find themselves when eventually discharged.

The sort of immobility problems covered in this chapter frequently give rise to one of the most difficult questions nurses have to answer, 'Will I be able to walk again?' Variations of this question are likely to be asked in the immediate aftermath of catastrophe as the patient or family seek hope that recovery will occur.

The nurse has to tread a tightrope. It would be easy to give encouraging answers and raise the patient's hopes of a full recovery. Such answers would be dishonest and cruel, and would lead to a demoralized patient never trusting a nurse again. Conversely, a bleak 'no' would destroy the patient and discourage them from attempting any rehabilitation. The truthful answer is that the nurse does not know, and neither does anybody else at this early stage.

Nurses should always be truthful with patients, and this is no exception to that rule. The way to deal with this sort of question, therefore, is to be honest but in an encouraging way, pointing out that it is too early to say how much recovery will occur, but that every effort will be made to ensure maximum progress. The nurse should also be realistic about the timescale involved; many months of hard work may be needed before any real improvement is made. Whatever happens, it is essential that the patient fighting to recover independence and self care ability should have a realistic view of the problems ahead and trust the staff who are trying to help.

References

Bobath B. (1980). *Look at it This Way: New Perspectives in Rehabilitation* (1980). Kent: Hodder and Stoughton with Open University Press.

Burke D., Murray D. (1975). *Handbook of Spinal Cord Medicine*. London: Macmillan.
Grundy D., Russell J., Swain A. (1986). A.B.C. of Spinal Cord Injury. London: *British Medical Journal*.
Kelly M. (1985). Loss and grief reactions as response to surgery. *Journal of Advanced Nursing*, No. 10, 517–525.
Parkes C.M. (1972). *Bereavement: Studies of Grief in Adult Life*. London: Tavistock.
Smith C. (1987). *Orthopaedic Nursing*. London: Heinemann.
Taggliacozzo D.L., Mauksch H. (1972). The patient's view of the patient's role. In *Patients, Physicians and Illness: A Source Book in Behavioural Science and Health* 2nd edn. New York: Free Press.
Walsh M. (1985). *Accident and Emergency Nursing: A New Approach*. London: Heinemann.

Bibliography

Buchanan L., Nawoczenski D. (1987). *Spinal Cord Injury*. Baltimore: Williams and Wilkins.
Hickey J. (1986). *Neurological and Neurosurgical Nursing*. Philadelphia: Lippincott.
Schoen D.C. (1986). *The Nursing Process in Orthopaedics*. Connecticut: Appleton-Century-Crofts.
Shergold L. (1986). Epidural and spinal anaesthetics. *Nursing Times*, 2nd July, 44–45.
Stewart J.D.M., Hallett J.P. (1983). *Traction and Orthopaedic Appliances*. Edinburgh: Churchill Livingstone.

7
Care of the child with a mobility problem

Orem's model of nursing recognizes the developmental dimension of patient care, and this is most clearly seen in considering the care of children. Children who have a mobility problem cannot just be held in a developmental limbo. Their emotional and social needs have to be met if they are in a hospital bed or being cared for at home in a hip spica. It is essential that those caring for them are aware of these developmental stages, so that any retardation due to a change in environment or circumstances will be recognized.

Piaget, a well known Swiss psychologist with particular interest in child development, described several stages that children go through to reach adolescence (Piaget, 1952). The first stage, which he named the sensorimotor stage, has particular reference to the immobile child as up to the age of two years the child is learning the relationship between the sensations that are felt and how the body can be moved. If the child is unable to move and make these experiments, to feel the world around him, the stage may be abnormally lengthened. Karn and Ragiel (1986) relate this stage to a time when the infant becomes aware of object permanences, such as the mother or a favourite toy. There will be signs of anxiety and panic if the parents go out of sight even for a short while, and the child will not be able to understand explanations that may be offered for their disappearance.

The second stage, which lasts until the child is about seven years, was referred to by Piaget as the pre-operational stage and is a time when the child can begin to use language and symbols. This provides nurses with a useful means of explaining treatments to a child by using pictures, another child as a model or a doll on which a plaster can be applied. As it is a time of language development, the child who is deprived of verbal stimulation will be retarded in this area. This is clearly of great importance in the hospitalized child. Ack (1983) suggests that it is a time when the child is most likely to perceive hospitalization as a punishment for misbehaviour. It is also a time when children frequently regress to bedwetting or to using 'baby language' to direct their carers attention to their feeling of loss – be it familiar surroundings or a mother who cannot stay.

By the age of about seven years, children have reached a stage of operational development when they can begin to form mental representations of a series of actions. Piaget refers to this as the concrete operational stage because, to perform this mental activity, the child has to use concrete objects – that is, objects with which the child is very familiar. Karn and Ragiel (1986) suggest that it is a time when the child's greatest fear is loss of control, and that anger and hostility to the staff and family will result when mobility is limited by orthopaedic equipment such as plaster casts or traction.

Once the child has reached the age of about twelve, there should be some indication that the formal operational stage has been reached. In this stage, the child should be able to follow through an idea with several variables of outcome, in other words engage in abstract, adult thought. In the ward situation, this may refer to the child being shown his X-rays and being told the options for treatment depending on the way healing of the fractures occurs.

Children who are immobilized for any length of time will have 'bottled up' energy with which they will have to come to terms. A common way for them to release it is by continually seeking the attention of carers in noisy, demanding behaviour. However, those children who shrink into their shell and become quiet and compliant are often overlooked in the general hubub of the ward, and it must not be forgotten that they have needs as well.

The child's need to play and explore the environment should not be left to chance. Even with the encumbrances of plasters such as a bilateral hip spica, children should be encouraged to move around on small trolleys and to meet ingroups with other children to maintain development of their socializing skills. Some hospitals employ play leaders to ensure that these immobile children have constructive play time; however, this tends to happen in specialist hospitals and certainly is not the norm in district general hospitals. It has been suggested that play is an outlet for the child's pent up anger and frustration, and as such the value of play cannot be underestimated.

All hospitals in which there are children with a mobility problem have a responsibility to ensure that the child's education does not suffer because of the time spent there. Obviously, no-one is suggesting that the child should be pressurized to study while they are unwell, in pain or suffering the after effects of hospital admission. However, most children will have times during their hospital stay when they will be able to continue with school work. Parents can help to provide a liaison with the child's school by taking school books into hospital so that the ward teacher will be able to offer some continuity. Schools programmes on the television are of great help and, as they are used by many schools as a method of teaching, they will also supply some continuity in the child's education. The ward teacher should be skilled in the teaching of hospitalized children, so that links are created between hospital and home. The aim is to ensure that when the child returns to school, the amount of work to be made up will be limited.

Ever since the Platt report in 1959, the position of the parent in the hospital ward has been safeguarded, in theory if not in practice. Every parent has a right to stay with their child, and every ward has the obligation to provide facilities for the parent. In some hospitals, this means a special bungalow or flat where parents can stay; in other hospitals, it means allowing parents to bring a caravan into the hospital grounds so that other children can come as well, thus keeping the family together. This can be essential in situations where the hospitalized child is critically ill and therefore likely to be in for some time.

A crucial factor in the child's progress is the attitude of ward staff to the presence of parents. McCallum (1983) has suggested that, when a child is admitted to hospital, it is important that as few barriers as possible are placed between child and parent. This should include educating parents in the more technical areas of the child's care so that they are able, for example, to blanket bath their child, even if he is in traction with a fractured femur. The parents should feel comfortable and not worry that they are doing anything wrong. In some cases, of course, it will include teaching a parent how to give various treatments to a child so that therapy can continue at home. This frequently applies to physiotherapy. In the case of a child with a mobility problem, it may mean teaching the parent how the child should climb stairs with crutches in safety, or it may include quadriceps exercises for the child to continue at home to increase knee stability.

This chapter will look at the care of the child in the same way as the three previous chapters have covered adult immobility problems. We will therefore start with problems of temporary mobility:
1. In a plaster of Paris cast
2. In traction
3. Following surgery
4. Due to fear and anxiety.

before looking at permanent mobility problems:
1. The child with a congenital handicap
2. The child with a mobility problem of sudden onset.

TEMPORARY MOBILITY PROBLEMS

Care of a child in a plaster of Paris splint

Because of the very nature of the way that they play and explore, children are prone to fractures and therefore to having a limb immobilized in plaster of Paris. This may be in the short term, as in the case of a greenstick fracture of the radius (four weeks), or for longer, as in the case of a child with a comminuted fracture of the lower third of tibia.

Whatever the reason for the plaster, once the child has become used to it and the original pain has decreased, possession of a plaster cast has a certain status and most children enjoy the attention.

When the plaster is first applied, the child should be

CARE OF THE CHILD WITH A MOBILITY PROBLEM

encouraged to move the fingers or toes to demonstrate to the staff that such movement is possible. The child may show a marked reluctance to do this in case it will be painful, and it may well be at first. The reasons for asking the child to move fingers and toes should be explained to the parents, as should the reasons for looking at the colour of the digits and checking sensation.

Limbs should always be raised for the first 24–48 hours. Following a difficult manipulation to oppose bone ends, when it is known that there will be substantial swelling, a longer period of elevation may be required. An upper limb may be raised in a roller towel or drawsheet suspended from an intravenous stand. If the patient is ambulatory, the limb should be placed in a high arm sling with the wrist above the elbow. When an above-elbow plaster has been applied, a broad arm sling should be used, ensuring that the hand is well supported by the edge of the sling.

For the child with a plaster on the lower limb, the need to raise the limb when sitting should be explained to the patient as well as to the parents or carers. The importance of checking the plaster for any cracks should be emphasized, especially around the back of the knee and the ankle where they are most likely to occur. Before any child with a lower leg plaster is able to leave hospital, whether following in-patient or out-patient treatment, a careful check must be made to ensure that the child is safe when mobile. Children think that walking with crutches is simple, but in fact it is an art that requires mastering. Patients should also be told exactly what signs to look for that will indicate that something has gone wrong inside the plaster. These signs will include swollen fingers or toes, a feeling of burning in one spot, any exudate from inside the plaster, a sudden offensive smell (this is a late sign and usually means that other signs have been ignored), or sudden pain in a limb that has been relatively pain-free. A card should be given to the parents reinforcing what they have been told about caring for the plaster and the limb following application of a cast.

An important point in teaching a child about their plaster is to do so in language that the child understands. This applies in general to all nursing care of children; the nurse must communicate on the same level as the child. The importance of work by Piaget and other child psychologists is vital in this area of nursing care.

All children with a cast enjoy collecting their friends' names on it, as well as jokes and other appropriate sentiments. However, friends should be discouraged from using watercolours to paint on the plaster as this can make it soggy and likely to disintegrate. Patients and parents should also be warned about getting the plaster wet when washing and can be guided into the careful use of polythene bags over the cast to keep it dry.

A child may be treated with a hip spica after surgery for congenital dislocation of the hip, or if they have sustained a facture of the femur. Hip spicas may be unilateral or bilateral (see Fig. 7.1) and usually extend from the nipple line to the

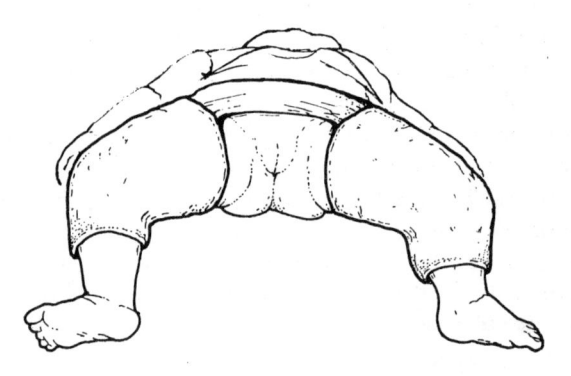

Fig. 7.1 A child in a bilateral hip spica. This particular plaster is sometimes referred to as a 'frog plaster' and may be used to treat children with congenital dislocation of the hip

ankle on the affected side. They may also include the foot on the affected side. Children, on the whole, adapt well to these plasters, although obviously the older the child the longer it will take to adapt. As these plasters are usually performed under general anaesthetic or heavy sedation, the child may be terrified on waking to find that movement of the lower limbs is impossible. As these children tend to be in the under-three age group, it is impossible to warn them before surgery about what the plaster will be like. On awakening, it is vital that a parent or someone very close to the child is at the bedside. It may be of help in overcoming the strangeness of it all if a favourite teddy bear or doll has had a similar plaster applied.

Children who are still in nappies should have the 'napkin' area of the plaster reinforced with some type of waterproof material, such as 'sleek', so that it does not become 'urine bogged'. Potty-trained children may have the occasional accidents when the plaster is first applied – this should be expected and allowed for. Boys frequently find difficulty in passing urine while in a hip spica, and it is sometimes necessary to hold them upright to mimic the position in which they are used to passing urine. As children quite often have difficulty in opening their bowels after a hip spica has been applied, this should be anticipated by including plenty of roughage in their diets and a high fluid intake. If this is not sufficient, a very mild aperient or paediatric glycerine suppository should be used. What must be prevented is constipation when the faeces become so hard that they are painful and cause the child a lot of avoidable anguish.

The child should be turned regularly from supine to prone to allow the plaster to dry completely and also to avoid pressure sores. Most children hate this at first until they feel secure with the member of staff doing it. Children appear instinctively to be able to tell if a nurse is unused to handling patients in such plasters, and this leads to feelings of insecurity and attempts to prevent the turning taking place. To turn a child in a hip spica requires two nurses or a nurse and a mother or visitor. The child should be lifted off the pillows to the edge of the bed, and the pillows rearranged to satisfy the new position. Thus, if turning from supine to prone, the pillows should be arranged in such a way that the child's chest is supported but there is no pillow under the face. Similarly, the legs should be supported but there should be room for the toes to move. If turning from prone to supine, there should be a pillow placed for the child's head and one under each foot. Once the pillows are in place, the arm should be positioned in such a way that the child is not lying on it after the turn. The patient is then turned towards the centre of the bed into the new position. There is some discussion about which way a child in a unilateral spica should be turned. It would appear that it does not really matter, as long as the spica is sound with no hint of cracks and provided that no undue pressure is put on it.

Once a child is happy in the spica, it is possible for a toddler to learn to mobilize themselves on a low trolley with castors. These are frequently made by fathers eager to help in a practical way. Most wards which care for such patients have an example of the type of trolley these can be. The only word of caution is that the children should not be able to leave the confines of the ward. Consideration should also be given to other children trying to learn to use crutches. A four-wheeled plaster hip spica can be potentially very dangerous in this situation!

Care of a child in traction

Children are frequently treated in skin traction for fractures of the femur and for supracondylar fractures of the humerus (Dunlop traction). Occasionally, children may be treated for a fractured femur with skeletal traction.

Gallows traction

Children aged two years or under who sustain a fractured shaft of femur are usually treated on Gallows (Bryant's) traction. Skin extensions are applied to the full length of both of the child's legs. To facilitate adhesion, the skin should be first sprayed with tincture of benzoin. It should also be confirmed that the child is not allergic to elastoplast. If the child has no known elastoplast allergies but has multiple other allergies, it might be as well to consider different forms of treatment. When applying the extensions, small nicks should be made in each edge so that the strapping moulds to the contours of the leg. This is especially important around the knee area. A crepe bandage should then be applied around each leg from the foot to the top of the thigh. The cord of the extensions may be used either singly or doubly to suspend the child from the overhead beam or from a pulley with sufficient weights to lift the buttocks off the bed (see Fig. 7.2). Whichever system is used it is vital that the buttocks remain off the bed for the traction to be effective. The advantage of tying the cords to the beam is that it prevents the child

CARE OF THE CHILD WITH A MOBILITY PROBLEM 141

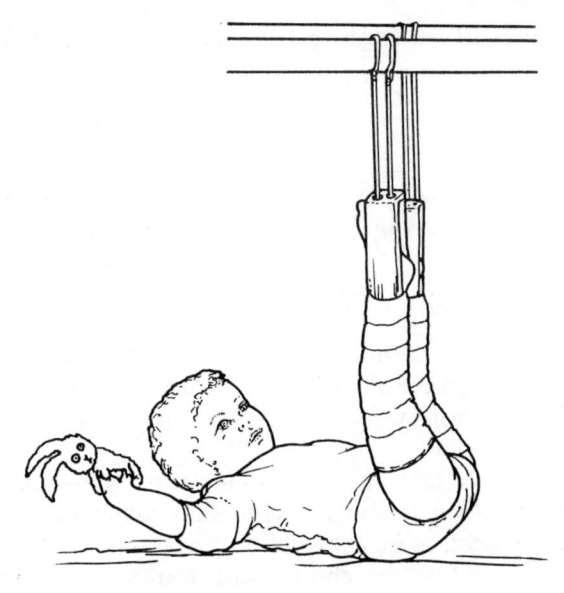

Fig. 7.2   *Gallows traction*

climbing out of the bed! This traction is usually applied either under a general anaesthetic or with the child under heavy sedation.

Once the traction has been applied, care of the child is aimed at ensuring that the traction continues to exert the required pull and that no complications of traction develop. In the first 24–48 hours, the child might experience severe muscle spasm and may require antispasmodic drugs. This will be obvious if the child suddenly cries out during sleep; in fact, the child can often be seen to 'jump'. In the early days, the child will also be fretful and in need of a lot of reassurance, usually best provided by the mother. However, most children adapt to this traction very quickly and are frequently quite happy in their 'upside down' world.

To ensure that the crepe bandages are not too tight, the child's pedal pulse should be checked, similarly every time the bandage is renewed, this pulse should be checked – hourly at first leading to four-hourly. Pressure sores are most likely to develop on the child's shoulders and the back of the head, and so these areas in particular should be carefully watched.

If a boy is old enough to have been toilet trained, he will often have problems passing urine into a urinal and will require a lot of patience both from the nursing staff and from parents.

This traction is not usually required for very long and the child may be nursed free in bed after four weeks although, as with all fractures, it depends on the X-ray appearance.

Fixed skin traction

This system of traction is used in the treatment of a fractured shaft of femur in an older child. It works on the principle of providing traction to fixed points within the Thomas' splint (see Fig. 7.3).

To apply this traction, the child has skin extensions applied to the affected leg as above. (As this is usually an older child, the leg may need to be shaved first.) Manual traction may be applied by holding the child's foot and gently pulling. The fracture site should be supported at all times. A crepe bandage is applied over the extensions and a correctly measured Thomas' splint is then applied. The cords from the extensions are tied onto the end of the splint as shown in Fig. 7.3. This forces the ring of the splint up into the child's groin and against the ischial tuberosity. As the cord has a certain amount of stretch in it, two tongue depressors should be strapped together, inserted into the cords and twisted in the manner of a windlass. A gamgee pad may be applied under the fracture site to maintain the anterior bow of the femur; also, any deformity may be corrected by placing gamgee in strategic positions. A crepe bandage may then be applied over the whole splint. This has the effect of slowing down the child's inquisitive fingers, and stops the extensions being peeled off to relieve boredom. The splint is then suspended from a pulley system, which will keep the leg elevated and allow the child to move up and down the bed with a certain amount of freedom. The amount of weight used should be balanced against the weight of the leg.

The nursing care of a child receiving this treatment will be aimed at preventing the development of complications from traction. One of the major problems is the development of pressure sores under the ring of the splint. Once the traction is

CARE OF THE CHILD WITH A MOBILITY PROBLEM 143

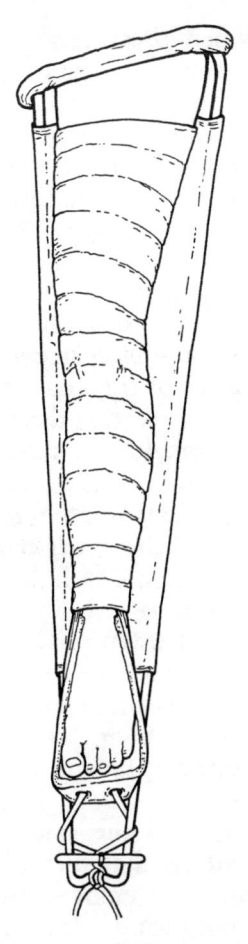

Fig. 7.3 *Fixed skin traction*

applied, the skin should be checked every two hours in the first instance for any signs of marking. The skin may be gently pulled from under the ring to check it, and this should be repeated all the way around the ring. If there is any sign of redness, the child's position should be altered to move the pressure-bearing area. If the child's skin is allowed to break down, the whole form of treatment may need altering. Some surgeons support the idea of applying a weight to the end of the splint to pull the ring away from the groin and relieve the pressure; others say that this reduces the effect of the traction.

The other areas where pressure sores may develop are over the achilles tendon from the edge of the supporting flannelette, and over the heel of the opposite foot which is frequently used to help push the child up the bed. Elbows also are at risk of becoming sore as they are frequently used as supports. Pressure on the common peroneal nerve as it wraps around the head of the fibula may develop if the leg is allowed to fall into external rotation and rest against the splint. This is shown by a loss of dorsiflexion.

As with all traction, the cords should be checked daily to ensure that they are running correctly over the pulleys and that there is no evidence of fraying.

The alternative way of treating this type of fracture is with sliding balanced traction. In this system, the cord from the extensions runs over a pulley with a weight hanging free. The weight is dependent on the size of the child and the pull needed to overcome the spasm of the quadriceps in the thigh. So that there is some counter traction from body weight, the foot of the bed should be raised.

Both of these types of traction allow the child to remain mobile within the confines of the bed and the traction cords. Once children are used to the traction, they can usually be persuaded to help in their own care by lifting themselves up for pressure area care and by moving the skin under the ring of the splint themselves.

Having become used to the traction, children are very secure in it, which means that they often become unhappy when it has to be removed. Removing two strips of elastoplast from a child's leg is not pleasant for the nurse or the patient. To facilitate this procedure, a brand of plaster remover could be used. The old adage of 'pull it off quickly – it won't hurt so much' is not strictly true because, if the plaster is pulled too fiercely, the superficial skin will be pulled off too and the child will have a sore leg. The traction should always be removed slowly and carefully. There should be a pause at each stage of the prodecure to allow the child to acclimatize to the new situation. Having waited several weeks to be able to get out of bed, many children are reluctant to mobilize. For some, it will take several days of patient handling by the physiotherapist and the nursing staff, during which the child will have to be taught to walk again.

Dunlop traction

This is one of the few forms of traction used on the upper limb. When they fall on an outstretched hand, children are at risk of sustaining a supracondylar fracture of the humerus. Because of the difficulty in maintaining the proximal fragment in the correct alignment, and the danger of damage to the brachial artery, this form of traction may be required.

Children's extensions are applied to the arm below the level of the fracture so that the spreader lies over the finger tips which should be extended. With the child lying flat, the arm should be brought out at right angles to the body and the cord from the extension placed over a pulley with an appropriate weight on the end of it. As the proximal fragment often 'cocks up' owing to the muscle attachment, a sling may be placed over the fragment with a weight hanging from it (see Fig. 7.4).

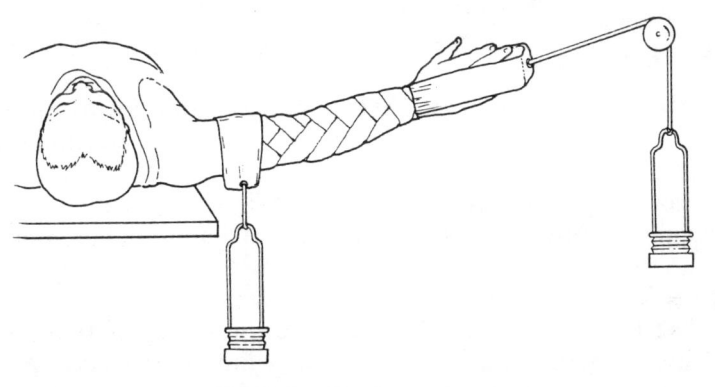

Fig. 7.4 *Dunlop traction*

To provide counter traction, the whole of one side of the bed (same side as injury) should be raised in a attempt to roll the child away from the affected arm. This position can be quite difficult to maintain as the tendency is for the child to creep over and nearer to the edge of the bed.

It is vitally important that the radial pulse is checked at half-hourly intervals when this traction is first applied to ensure that there is no embarrassment of the circulation to the hand. While the child is in this traction, hand exercises to the affected hand should be encouraged.

Care of a child with mobility problems following surgery

Following even relatively minor surgery, most children will require a period of immobilization to recover from the anaesthetic or the stress of undergoing an operation. The length of time that the child is immobilized and the degree of immobilization depends on the surgery performed and how the child feels within himself.

The reasons why a child may be immobile are similar to those in an adult, that is:

1. Pain
2. Intravenous infusions
3. Wound drains
   and, in addition:
4. Fear and anxiety.

The child in pain

The way in which children exhibit the pain they feel, and the way in which that behaviour is interpreted, is a complex matter. In the very young child, it is often assumed that they do not feel pain as acutely as adults and therefore require less analgesia. However, research has shown that a child as young as a few months old will withdraw their limbs from painful stimuli.

The reasons why children react so differently to pain are many. It is suggested that children see a link between pain and punishment and will search for a reason for their punishment. It has also been suggested that, following a punishment, many parents are overcome with guilt and lavish the child with signs of love and affection. If these are the only times that the child is shown these signs of love, the child may even enjoy the pain and punishment because they know it will be followed by lavish tokens of love.

The pressure on a child to act out the role stereotype in response to pain may be great. Therefore, a boy may be under a great deal of pressure not to show 'sissy' emotions but to act 'like a man'. If the pain is too great and the boy does cry, not only does he have his pain to contend with but also the fear of letting the side down and not living up to expectations. Girls,

CARE OF THE CHILD WITH A MOBILITY PROBLEM   *147*

on the other hand, are expected to show their feelings and do not associate crying with a feeling of 'giving in'.

When assessing the child in pain, these background influences must be taken into account so that, regardless of what the nurse feels about the severity of the child's pain, the patient has nursing interventions appropriate for the degree of pain that is demonstrated.

How a child tells of the severity of the pain felt has always been a problem. Very young children find it difficult to express pain and may use words such as 'hot' to describe a painful area. Other children may not be able to verbalize their pain, but their general restlessness and the way they hold the painful part will be indicative. Yet others will become withdrawn and depressed but be unable to explain why.

Mather and Mackie (1983) looked at postoperative pain and found that 75% of children complained of pain on the day of operation. Of those children the ones who were prescribed controlled and non-controlled drugs, the non-controlled drugs were given exclusively. The researchers also found that the doses given were either too small or too infrequent to be of any real benefit to the patient. To try to overcome this problem of inappropriate drugs being given at inappropriate times, Baker and Wong (1987) developed the 'QUEST' notion: this may be explained as follows:

Question the child. Emphasize the positive elements of behaviour rather than the negative.

Use a pain scale. Some children will be able to use a pain thermometer and gauge the severity of their pain on a scale of 1–10. Other children may be able to use a faces value scale in which there are six small faces, each with a different expression indicating 'no pain at all' at the one extreme to 'hurts as much as possible' at the other. This last face should have tears as well as an unhappy expression (see Fig. 7.5).

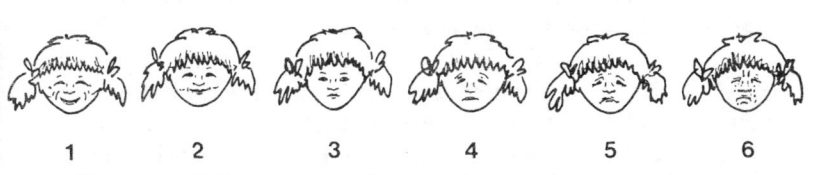

Fig. 7.5 *A face pain scale – to be used as an aid when assessing a child's pain*

Evaluate the behaviour. Observation of behaviour is a valuable way of assessing the efficacy of the nursing intervention, especially in the very young child. One way in which a young child may demonstrate pain is by shouting 'I hate you' or 'get out of here', whereas a school-age child may have learned to describe pain such as 'throbbing', 'terrible', or 'torture'.

Sensitize parents. This includes involving parents in the assessment of the child's behaviour; after all, they usually know the child and the child's reaction to pain better than anyone else. Baker and Wong suggest that parents should be taught about the various types of behaviour that children may exhibit when they are in pain.

Take action. This will include giving the correct medication at the correct time interval to give the child continuous pain relief. However, it also includes taking other actions to promote the child's comfort and feeling of well-being, such as helping the child into a comfortable position and rubbing the painful area. Some children find it helpful if they are told the exact nature of the pain and the cause of it, but only if this is done in language and concepts that the child can understand.

By using this system of assessing the child's pain and then acting on the assessment, it is suggested that the child will feel less pain, that they will not exhibit behaviour indicative of an attempt to cope with severe pain, and that there will be no evidence of the altered physiology of pain such as tachycardia, dilated pupils and hyperventilation.

When the child's pain is brought down to tolerable levels, the level of mobility will be increased. Both the nurse and the physiotherapist will find improved cooperation of the child in walking the required distances, breathing deeply to ward off chest infections, and performing specific exercises to improve muscle power and joint stability.

The child with an intravenous infusion

Most children find the setting up of intravenous infusions horrific and painful. Once they are in place and running well, however, children are either worried by them and reluctant to let anyone or anything come near them, or they are consumed with curiosity and continually pull at the covering bandages and strapping to look at them. Intravenous infusions are also a great status symbol among children.

Children should be told exactly why they have an infusion – but again in language and using ideas that they can understand. A young child will find this very difficult to grasp. Children should also be told what it will feel like if something goes wrong; for example, the arm will become hot and painful and will look red, the drip will stop dropping at a regular rate, or the dressing and the bandage will become wet.

To preserve the infusion and avoid subjecting the child to multiple attempts at cannulating veins, the cannula should be well fixed in place, first with a specific small dressing, such as Velafix, and then with more substantial strapping (having first ensured that there is no allergy). Finally, a crepe bandage should cover the whole area – over a splint if the cannula has been inserted at a joint – and the ends strapped down.

As children recover, the problem lies not so much in persuading them to be more mobile, but rather in limiting their mobility! While the intravenous infusion is in place, the child should be told exactly how mobile he or she can be and what behaviour is not acceptable. Most children react well if they can see the fairness of what they are being told and the reasons behind it, rather than merely having a strict list of rules dictated to them without rhyme or reason.

The child with a wound drain

Children are more likely to accept the presence of wound drains if they are told the reason for the drains and the limits within which they can move. To facilitate this acceptance of drains, nursing staff should ensure that the drain is well anchored to the patient so that there is no 'drag' on the drain site. The connections should also be checked to ensure that there is no likelihood of it separating. Suddenly seeing a large blood stain on their clothes which will reduce patients' confidence in the nursing staff and upset them considerably. If the sight of blood-stained fluid in the drainage bottle upsets the child, it could be placed in a paper bag to camouflage it. Children with drains which require gravity rather than suction need careful explanations about why the collecting bottle must always be lower than the wound site.

There is no reason why a child with a wound drain should not mobilize within the limits of the recovery time and ability. However, nurses should be aware that what is an everyday occurrence for them is a once-in-a-lifetime situation for others. Children especially are unlikely to have any experience of the limitations imposed on them by such appendages as drains or infusions, and they will require careful, repeated assurances and information about what they can and cannot do.

When children are recovering, the frustrated energy they may feel at their immobility will need to be redirected into more positive and useful outlets. Sometimes, children can help by stamping charts for the ward staff or making decorations for the ward. It must be recognized that 'bad behaviour' usually has a reason and every effort should be made to find the cause, for the benefit of the child and staff alike!

Care of the child who is immobile due to anxiety and fear

To reduce a child's fear and anxiety postoperatively, preparation should commence before admission. Even those children who are admitted to hospital as an emergency will be better prepared if they feel secure with their parents. If the child has learnt that hospitals are positive places where people try to help others to get better, there will be less fear of admission. However, if the child has been threatened with hospital as a punishment for bad behaviour in the past, hospitalization will not easily be accepted. To add to the upset, the child will be trying to see what he or she has done to deserve such punishment.

Similarly, children who have only slept in one bed, with a very set routine, a light in a particular place etc., will have difficulty settling into any strange environment let alone a hospital ward at a time when they are feeling ill and vulnerable.

There are many children's books available which will help prepare a child for admission to hospital, some produced commercially and some produced by such organizations as the National Association of the Welfare of Children in Hospital (NAWCH). Some junior schools now organize a visit of NAWCH to the school so that their pupils are aware of what a stay in hospital might entail. Similarly, some hospitals arrange for visits from local school children to show them the inside of a hospital. The *Which Report* (1980) showed that children who are prepared for hospital will settle in quicker, cooperate with the staff better and, consequently, have a shorter length of stay.

For children having planned surgery, some hospitals organize a pre-admission afternoon when the children can visit the ward into which they will be admitted and meet the staff and some of the children who will be admitted at the same time as themselves. At this afternoon, the children may also play with dolls dressed in appropriate uniforms with a play leader who can help the children to 'act out' some of the procedures that they will see and experience as a patient. Even the well-prepared child will feel vulnerable and frightened postoperatively. Because of this, there may be a genuine reluctance to move and an insistence on lying rigidly in one position. For such a child, the complications which may develop include pressure sores, chest infections and depression. Children who are reluctant to mobilize in any way postoperatively should be encouraged to explain to the nursing staff why they feel that way. This they may do through their mother or directly to the nurse; for this to happen the child must feel that the nurse has time, is interested and is able to help. Therefore, it is up to the nursing staff to create such an atmosphere within the ward. If and when the nurse can establish why the child feels unable to move, steps must be taken to overcome the problem. Helping the child to become mobile following surgery should not be the result of constant nagging from the staff and parents, but should happen as a result of the child overcoming the fear and anxiety and thus feeling able and confident to start mobilizing again.

PERMANENT MOBILITY PROBLEMS

Congenital mobility problems

Children may have a congenital mobility problem due to a defect in the development of the nervous system or to a mechanical problem such as congenital talipes equinovarus (club foot) or congenital absence of a bone in the lower leg.

Whatever the type of handicap, the children must be allowed to develop to their full potential to enable them, where possible, to take their place as active members of society.

Children with both mental and physical handicaps are usually cared for in the community, while only those with very severe mental handicap remain in the institutional setting of a hospital.

Mobility problems due to neural maldevelopment

Because muscles, like all body tissues, are dependent on the nervous system to act as a control mechanism, malfunction at certain points of the nervous system will be reflected in the child's lack of motor skills. If the defect is in the brain, as in children with cerebral palsy, there will be a spastic paralysis similar to that following a cerebrovascular accident or head injury. The reason for the spasticity is that the spinal reflexes are still intact but are not controlled by the cerebrum. In this instance, there is frequently a mental handicap as well.

Cerebral palsy

Cerebral palsy manifests itself in a symmetrical or an asymmetrical disability. The symmetrical form frequently follows an inherited pattern with a one in four recurrence risk. For those families with a child with an asymmetrical cerebral palsy, the recurrence rate is less than one in two hundred.

Children with an asymmetrical cerebral palsy (hemiplegia) will need to be reminded of the affected side at all times as they frequently forget its presence. Thus, when teaching a child to dress, the affected limb should always be dressed first; at meal times, the affected limb should always be placed on the table within the child's vision and, if possible, a padded spoon provided to try to encourage the use of the implement by the affected hand with the grip reflex. Every effort should be used to promote the child's awareness of the affected arm.

For a child with cerebral palsy to be mobile, both legs and feet must be stable enough to weight-bear. Once the child starts standing, great emphasis must be placed on the position of the foot on the ground as these children frequently have an equinus deformity. In an attempt to correct this, the child may wear a below-knee caliper which will allow concentration on other parts of the gait. However, if the use of an appliance fails to correct the problem, an operation to lengthen the calcaneal tendon may be performed. This will allow the child's heel to be brought down to the ground and reduce the amount of toe walking. Sometimes, in children with hemiplegic cerebral palsy, the affected leg is shorter than the other one. Those with a shortening of more than 1.25 cm usually have a raise put on their shoe to facilitate walking and standing.

Diplegia is a form of cerebral palsy in which all four limbs are affected, although the legs are affected more than the arms. Characteristically, the muscles are hypertonic and there is an abundance of unwanted, uncontrolled movements. Once the child starts to stand, the aim is for the child to develop a broad-based, stable gait. This may be quite difficult as, in these children, there is a strong tendency for the hips to flex and adduct. It is generally thought that the use of walking aids such as rollators should not be encouraged as these only increase the degree of hip flexion because the children tend to take their weight through their arms. Great care should be taken to prevent the development of fixed flexion deformities of the hip and knee, especially before the child starts walking.

Two particular approaches in the treatment of children with cerebral palsy have been specially recognized among the many forms of treatment available. These are:

1. The Bobath method, in which the emphasis is on inhibition of the reflexes as these according to Bobath and Bobath (1980), are responsible for the major difficulties children with cerebral palsy experience in mobilization.
2. Conductive education developed by Dr Andras Peto, in which the child with cerebral palsy has to learn and relearn patterns of movement. The child is first encouraged to say what they intend to do, followed by what they are doing while actually performing the movement.

Spina bifida

This is a condition of malformation of the vertebrae which may or may not affect the spinal cord. There are three main types of spina bifida (see Fig. 7.6):

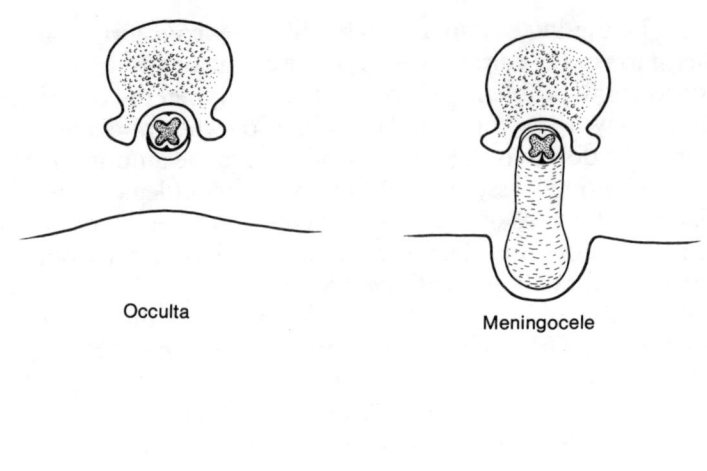

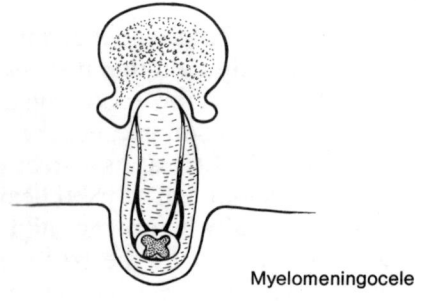

Fig. 7.6 *The three degrees of spina bifida*

1. Spina bifida occulta, in which there is a failure of fusion of the vertebral arch in one vertebra, usually in the lumbar region.
2. Meningocele, which is fairly uncommon (4% of cases according to McCarthy, 1984) and represents a defect in the vertebral arch and formation of a sac containing cerebrospinal fluid by the meninges. The skin over the area is usually intact.
3. Myelomeningocele, in which the spinal cord and all nerve roots lie outside the vertebral canal.

The types of spina bifida fall into two distinct categories. In the first type there is a complete loss of spinal cord function below the lesion (flaccid paralysis and sensory loss). The second type is associated with loss of the corticospinal tracts but there is preservation of some reflex activity (a very small group of patients have a hemimyelomeningocele in which one leg is normal but the other is affected).

There cannot be any realistic speculation about the ability of the child to walk independently until the age of about two years. At this stage, the child should be trying to stand, and there should be some assessment of the type of orthosis that will be required to aid standing and walking. For the child with a high lesion, a pelvic or thoracic band will be required for support together with a rollator; the child learns to walk by swivelling weight from one leg to the other. Eventually, the child learns to use crutches and a 'jump to' gait pattern. The advantages of encouraging the child at least to stand are thought to lie in the improvement of circulation to the legs and in kidney function. However, it is recognized that those who require substantial orthoses will revert eventually to using a wheelchair rather than persevering with walking. It is vital that children who use wheelchairs are taught to transfer themselves in and out of the wheelchair, and also are given arm strengthening exercises so that they can maintain as much self care as possible.

As some children with spina bifida have a sensory loss in the limbs, they must be taught the importance of regularly looking for any signs of pressure on their skin. This is especially important if orthoses are used which have very firm parts and pieces of metal that can severely damage the skin.

Immobility due to a mechanical problem

This heading covers congenital abnormality affecting the mechanics of mobility rather than muscular control. The impact of these problems has been reduced over the years as a result of children being examined within a few days of birth and any treatment started very early. For many, the criterion is to correct the deformity before the child commences walking so that poor gait and balance, can be prevented.

Congenital talipes equino varus

This condition of the foot and ankle used to be blamed on poor fetal position, but it is more likely to result from an ideopathic muscle imbalance or a muscle imbalance due to spina bifida. The deformity itself is a plantar flexion of the ankle joint, inversion of the subtalar joint and adduction of the midtarsal joint (Powell, 1986) (see Fig. 7.7). The im-

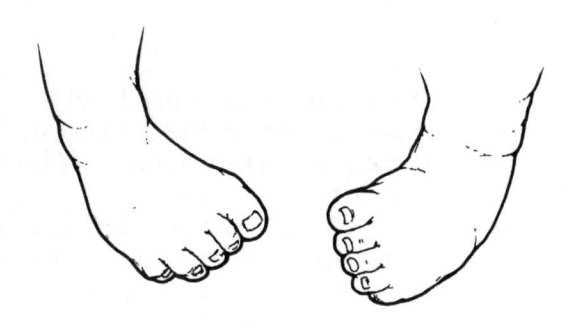

Fig. 7.7 *Talipes equinovarus or 'club foot', in which the small, underdeveloped heel is higher than the forefoot*

mediate treatment is stretching the foot into an over-corrected position. If it reverts to the deformity, the foot should be held in the over-corrected position using strapping or plaster bootees which extend over the flexed knee in an effort to stop the baby kicking them off.

If the deformity is not correctable in this way due to a short calcaneal tendon or to soft tissues on the medial side, the tendon may be surgically lengthened and the soft tissue released to allow the correct position to be reached.

If the deformity is still present when the child starts walking, surgery on the lateral aspect of the foot (wedge arthrodesis of the calcaneum/cuboid) may be performed.

Amelia and dysmelia: absence of a limb or part of a limb

The cause of this condition is unknown except for the well-known thalidamide cases. In a very small number, a familial pattern can be detected. Lower limb deficiencies alone account for only 14% of all cases, indicating that the majority of instances involve the upper limbs.

The commonest upper limb deficiency is absence of one hand and two thirds of the forearm. There is frequently evidence of tiny digit buds at the distal end of the limb. Children should start wearing a light weight prosthesis from the age of six months to familiarize them with its presence. By the age of $3\frac{1}{2}$–4 years, a myo-electric prosthesis may be used, in which two electrodes connect with the flexor and extensor muscles to produce movement of the fingers in the prosthesis. These hands are powered by rechargeable batteries which add to the overall weight of the prosthesis.

Children with amelia develop an unusual degree of flexibility of the hip joint and control of the feet to compensate for their lack of a hand and arm.

The most common form of dysmelia in the lower limb is shortening of a long bone. Congenital absence of fibula is usually accompanied by a short, bowed tibia and a small, everted foot. For these children, an extension prosthesis may be fitted at the end of the first year to familiarize the child with the weight. If a prosthesis is to be fitted successfully, the foot needs to be in extreme plantar flexion. If there is limited shortening (less than 10 cm), consideration must be given to amputating the foot in order to obtain a good cosmetic effect.

In most cases of femoral dysmelia, it is the proximal part of the bone that is absent while the distal part and the rest of the limb are normal. When the hip is stable, an extension prosthesis may be applied with the weight being taken through the ischial tuberosity. For those children with an unstable hip, a prosthesis with a pelvic band and buttock support will be required.

Children with a limb deficiency need to be encouraged to put all remaining joints through a full range of movement to maintain their mobility. Those with absent or short lower limbs will find balancing to sit very difficult and may require extra supports in the early days of sitting to help them learn balance. As many children with this condition will not be able to play in the usual accepted way, they should be encouraged to explore their surroundings using their limbs or limb buds in whatever way they can. Learning to walk can be a long drawn out procedure with many falls on the way. Children should be allowed to carry on, although they should be prevented from seriously injuring themselves.

Emotional development of children with a congenital handicap

Handicap is defined by the United Nations, after the World Health Organization, as 'a function of the relationship between disabled persons and their environment. . . . Handicap is the loss or limitation of opportunities to take part in life of the community on an equal level with others' (Stopford, 1987).

Relationships between the handicapped child and the environment depend, as with any other child, on the bonding process with the mother and experiences with the immediate environment. The arrival of a handicapped child within a family will immediately place added stress on family dynamics. How the family adapt to this stress will influence the way in which the affected child sees his or her place within the family which, after all, is the first social unit that most are involved with. A child's first ideas about his or her own importance will be developed from this integration within the family. Because the desire to protect her child is probably greater when the child is handicapped, mothers of such children may make the child's transition to socializing in the wider world more difficult. Very young handicapped children are often accepted relatively easily as people expect young children to be dependent and not in full control of themselves. However, as the child becomes older, differences between the handicapped and non-handicapped child become greater, and the handicapped child may begin to experience the first feelings of being different.

Many children enjoy the feeling of security within their own family but when they venture into the outside world have these positive feelings confused by the negative influences of others. This may lead to depression and aggression in the child (Stopford, 1987). While the handicapped child is developing a role within the family, the needs of other children must also be met. Each member of the family must have a complementary role which harmonizes with the others. When the expectations of each other's role fail to materialize, there is disharmony in the home.

Children with relatively minor handicaps may attend conventional local authority schools, which has the advantage of integrating the handicapped and non-handicapped. This is seen by many as the place where integration should start. For children with a mental handicap, the integration in class may not be so easy, as the educational needs of the majority will take precedence. A compromise might be to separate the children for some classes, although during play and meal times, and in certain non-academic classes, integration may take place.

The transition to secondary school may be more difficult as children tend to move around more between classes. However, if the problems are met with enthusiasm within the school, they can often be overcome. The child's wishes should be the most important factor in the choice of school. Anderson and Clarke (1982) suggest that handicapped teenagers tend to be rather isolated, both at special schools and at ordinary schools, and have a problem relating to others. This problem of developing relationships would appear to be even worse outside the school. In the same study, Anderson and Clarke showed that 30–60% of handicapped teenagers had no friends outside school. Dorner (1976) showed that 40% of teenagers with spina bifida had no friends outside school or college. The reasons for this are given by Dorner as lack of opportunity, shyness, low self-esteem, problems of mobility and specific unacceptable handicaps, such as incontinence and speech impairments which reduce communication. The loneliness and unhappiness felt by these youngsters create a self-fulfilling prophecy as they become less attractive to others because of their unhappiness.

Adolescence is a time of great change and adjustment for all youngsters; for those who are handicapped, the problems of readjustment are even greater. Teenagers are naturally preoccupied with their own appearance, and the need to conform with the demands placed on them by society and the media is very great. The conflict this causes handicapped adolescents can be seen even in such basic areas as a continued dependence on another person to visit a toilet, get in a car or cut up food in a restaurant. This dependence will affect their self-esteem and may also cause them to turn to their disability and adopt a 'sick role'. This may be their way of dealing with the stigma they may feel as a result of interaction with other youngsters.

It is at adolescence that the first sexual experimentation

takes place amongst youngsters. For the handicapped, this may prove very difficult if, even after overcoming the problems of meeting others, over-protective parents will not give them the 'space' to experience these situations. The chances of a non-handicapped teenager developing a relationship with a handicapped teenager must be reduced by fear of ridicule and the attitudes of others, not least both sets of parents. Greengross (1976) suggests that non-handicapped teenagers gain their sexual information from their peers, unlike handicapped teenagers who gain their sexual knowledge from parents, schools or residential institutions. This suggests that the content of their information will be very different because of the difference in sources. Any sexual counselling that handicapped people may have must include the physical effect that their handicap may have on their own sexual performance. This should include maintaining an erection and ejaculation in the male, and being able to enjoy clitoral and/or vaginal orgasm in the female. It must also include the differences between themselves and non-handicapped individuals, so that there can be an appreciation of each other's needs. Contraception is a subject that may be avoided if pregnancy is thought unlikely. However, for any adolescent girl, accurate information about what will make her pregnant and how to avoid it is important – for the handicapped teenager, it is crucial. Dorner suggests that many handicapped youngsters reach adulthood with only the vaguest idea of what contraception entails. For those who have a genetically transmitted condition, frank discussion with a genetic counsellor is essential so that the likelihood of the handicap being passed on is understood and nothing is left to chance.

The development of groups such as PHAB (physically handicapped and able-bodied) has given both handicapped and non-handicapped youngsters a chance to meet together and begin to break down the barriers between 'normal and abnormal'. However, it remains a sad fact that, frequently, the attitude of adults is transferred to their children, and the use of such terms as 'spastic' and 'mongol' become terms of abuse.

SUMMARY

As was mentioned at the beginning of this chapter, the needs of the immobile child are different from those of adults and should be met in a different way. The child should be assessed as a child and not as a small adult, and consideration must be given to their stage of development as this will influence their understanding of any situation. Due consideration must also be given to the family so that, more than in any other branch of nursing, there is care of the whole family and not just one individual. At all times, the nurse must understand that children think in different ways from adults and therefore be prepared to see things through the child's eyes if she is to care effectively for that child. Orem's emphasis on the developmental dimension of self care is crucial in planning care for the child with mobility problems.

References

Ack M. (1983). Psychological effects of illness, hospitalization and surgery. *Children's Health Care*, 11, 132–136.

Anderson E., Clarke L. (1982). *Disability in Adolescence*. London: Methuen.

Baker C., Wong D. (1987). QUEST: a process of pain assessment in children. *Orthopaedic Nursing*, 6 (1), 11–20.

Bobath B., Bobath B. (1980). *Rehabilitation of a Child with Cerebral Palsy. Look At It This Way: New Perspectives in Rehabilitation*. Kent: Hodder and Stoughton with Open University Press.

Dorner S. (1976). Psychological and social problems of families of adolescent spina bifida: A Preliminary Report. *Developmental Medicine and Child Neurology*, 15, Supplement 29, 24–27.

Eland J.M. (1977). Children's communication of pain. In *Pain: A source Book for Nurses and Other health Professionals*, (Jacox A., ed.). Boston: Little, Brown and Co., – .

Greengross W. (1976). *Entitled to Love*. London: Malaby Press in Association with National Fund for Research into Crippling Diseases.

Karn M., Ragiel C. (1986). The psychological effects of immobilisation in the paediatric orthopaedic patient. *Orthopaedic Nursing*, 5 (6).

McCarthy G., ed. (1984). *The Physically Handicapped Child*. London: Faber and Faber.

McCallum A.T. (1983). The chronically ill child: A guide for parents and professionals. *Child Today*, 11 (5), 36.

Mather L., Mackie J. (1983). The incidence of postoperative pain in children. *Pain*, 15, 271–282.

Piaget J. (1952). *The Origins of Intelligence in Children*. New York: International Universities Press.

Powell M. (1986). *Orthopaedic Nursing*. Edinburgh: Churchill Livingstone.

Smith C. (1987). *Orthopaedic Nursing*. London: Heinemann.

Stark G.D. (1977). *Spina Bifida*. Oxford: Blackwell Scientific Publications.

Stopford V. (1987). *Understanding Disability, Causes, Characteristics and Coping*. London: Edward Arnold.

Bibliography

Brechin A., Liddiard P., Swain J. (1983). *Handicap in a Social World*. Kent: Hodder and Stoughton with Open University Press.

Jukes J., Russell S., Stapley R. (1983). Coping with handicap. *Nursing (Oxford)*, 2 (20), 586–589.

Steele S., ed. (1977). *Nursing Care of the Child with a Long-term Illness*. Connecticut: Appleton-Century-Crofts.

Stiff B. (1985). Adolescence and physical handicap. *Nursing (Oxford)*, 2 (40), 1192–1194.

8
The immobile individual in the community

The emphasis on moving patients out of the hospital setting has led to changes in the care available in the community. In all areas of care, the large institutions have been replaced by small community homes, and the habit of keeping patients in hospital for months on end has been replaced by the philosophy of early discharge to the care of the community service.

This chapter will look at:
1. The preparation of the patient in hospital or an institution for a move into the community.
2. The facilities available in the community for those with a mobility problem.
3. The financial aid and support available in the community for those with a mobility problem.

PREPARATION OF THE PATIENT FOR TRANSFER INTO THE COMMUNITY

One of the main advantages of using Orem's model of nursing is seen to be the total commitment to the patient eventually being self caring. In the model, this is the goal for all care and, if successful, it overcomes the situation where today the patient is sitting in hospital as the passive recipient of care and tomorrow he or she is helped out of the ambulance and left to cope on their own.

Preparation for self care involves 'rehabilitation', which ideally should start the moment the patient is admitted.

Throughout their training, nurses are encouraged to be the 'doers' of care. Even the attitude of many patients is that they are in hospital to be cared for to the exclusion of doing anything for themselves. There are many subtle reasons for this which encompass not only people's attitude to care in hospital, but also their attitude to their own responsibility for their health. Some would argue that, by providing a 'free' health service, we have removed the individual's responsibility to care for his or her own health. When people have to pay directly for their health care, they may appear to be more aware of their own health needs.

If the care that nurses give in hospital is to be relevant and in the patient's best interests, it must emphasize the need for the patient, eventually, to care for themselves and/or be cared for by significant others at home. This should be a gradual transition, not a sudden overnight change and, for this to occur, care given in hospital must be with a self care goal in sight. No-one would suggest that every patient will eventually care for themselves, and for many self care involves the active participation of family and significant others. Those for whom total self care is not a realistic goal must be assessed in that light, and the level of self care that is appropriate aimed for, the deficit being made good by the community nursing service and other agencies.

If the preparation for discharge into the community is to start as soon as possible after the patient's admission, the goals of care must be patient-centred and not nurse-centred. A simple example of this is patients maintaining their own standards of personal hygiene. Nurses traditionally think that all patients should have a bath every day. For many people, bathing occurs once or twice a week, and for some, far less frequently than that. A nurse-centred goal may be to ensure that the patient has a bath every day, yet the patient may normally manage with a strip wash twice a week. Which goal is the more realistic and relevant for that patient's self care at home, and also the more readily attainable?

For patients whose mobility problems will continue after their discharge and, in some cases, for the rest of their lives, preparation for discharge must ensure that their mobility is appropriate for the type of accommodation into which they are being discharged. Sometimes, the use of distances in the ward may be totally unrealistic in comparison with what the patient will find at home. A goal such as 'able to walk to the bathroom to wash' may be attainable on the ward, but what about the flight of stairs that have to be negotiated in the patient's home?

Patients who have a mobility problem within the confines of the bed may be actually unable to get out of a high hospital bed. Again, whether or not they can achieve this is unrealistic if, when they get home, their bed is a low divan which will not pose the same problem. In hospital, the difficulty may be overcome by the use of adjustable height 'hi-lo' beds, as long as the nursing staff remember to leave the bed low enough to enable the patient to get out of it.

Hospitals which specialize in caring for patients with mobility problems often have rehabilitation units into which the patients can be transferred before their discharge home. These units may have fewer nursing staff but have a greater occupational therapist/physiotherapist input than other wards. Again, the nurse's role will be seen much more clearly as an educator or facilitator rather than a 'doer' of nursing care. This type of nursing role is often much easier to define in such a unit than it is in a general ward.

Patients requiring specific walking aids on discharge will need to be entirely safe with them in the many situations in which they are likely to find themselves. For example, while patients may seem able to manoeuvre their elbow crutches sufficiently well to return home to a flat or bungalow with no stairs, they must also be able to negotiate steps, the pavement curb, or to climb onto a bus, if they are not to be rendered housebound.

Care in rehabilitating a patient, be it in the ward soon after admission or in a rehabilitation unit, should reflect a multi-disciplinary approach as the distinct roles of the nurse, occupational therapist and physiotherapist become less obvious and 'merge at the edges'. In the past, health professionals have been guilty of guarding their own area of patient care and of working in isolation. It was thought that the introduction of the nursing process and care plans would enable their use by all disciplines as workable strategies reflecting all aspects of care. In some of the more forward-looking areas this happens, but in a majority of hospitals the care plans are still seen as the property of the nursing staff for their exclusive use. There is clearly a danger that, unless nurses adopt a 'hands off' self care philosophy, they will undo the good work of staff such as occupational therapists and physiotherapists in preparing the patient for the reality of self care in the community.

There are specific mobility skills that patients may need to acquire before they can be self caring at home. These skills fall into the broad categories considered below.

Walking skills

1. With one stick
2. With two sticks
3. With crutches
4. Using a walking frame.

Teaching someone to walk again in hospital usually involves the physiotherapist working with the patient both in the ward area and in the physiotherapy department. If the care that the nurse gives the patient is to be consistent, she must be aware of the principles by which the physiotherapist works so that they can be continued when the physiotherapist is not on the ward.

Before walking can commence, the patient must be able to stand and balance. To help the patient achieve this, an aid may be required – as a principle, the wider the base of the aid and the weight-bearing area, the more stable the patient will be. In practice, this means that a frame with weight-bearing on both feet will provide a wider base than two sticks and standing on one leg. The other principle is that the higher the patient takes the weight, the more stable the patient will be. Thus, patients who walk with axillary crutches will be more stable than those with elbow crutches. Similarly, a chest-high gutter frame will provide more stability than the usual waist-high walking frame. On the other hand, walking sticks provide the least stability.

Once mobilization commences, every effort must be made to help the patient establish an acceptable gait pattern rather than a disjointed series of hops.

When walking with a frame, the patient should be encouraged to lift the frame to arms length, set it down and walk into it (see Fig. 8.1). Inevitably, the patient will be taught in several stages at first, but the overall aim should still be that of establishing a pattern. When a rollator is used (a frame on wheels), the patient can be taught to walk with a more flowing pattern because foot movement occurs without having to stop to move the frame.

When using crutches, it is important that the patient takes as much weight as possible on the wrists and arms, rather than the axillae. This gives more control. Walking with crutches involves either a three- or four-point gait, the term 'point' referring to the number of weight-bearing areas that touch the ground. There is some discrepancy about whether feet together or crutches together count as one point or two, but it is assumed here that if four points actually touch the floor it is a four-point gait (see Fig. 8.2).

If both feet can weight-bear, one of two patterns of gait may be used – either both crutches can be put about 18 inches in front of the toes and then both feet swung forward 18 inches in front of the crutches, or alternatively, one crutch can be moved forward at the same time as the opposite foot, followed by the remaining crutch and foot. Although this sounds awkward, it can become a quite natural way of walking. Two sticks can be used in much the same way, although as the weight-bearing is lower (i.e. at the hand rather than in the axilla), it will not be so stable.

Stick walking is used when patients can take more weight through the feet than those using crutches. It is also used to give some confidence to patients who are a little unsteady by providing them with a wider base.

When measuring a patient for the correct size of walking aid, the following points are important:
1. Sticks. Measure the distance between the patient's ulnar styloid process and the heel. If this is done while the patient is lying in bed, an inch must be added to allow for the heel on the shoe.
2. Axillary crutches. Measure the hand grip as for the walking sticks. The axillary pad should to be two inches (three fingers) below the patient's axilla. If the patient takes too much weight through the axilla, there is a danger of injury to the brachial plexus.

168 MOBILITY

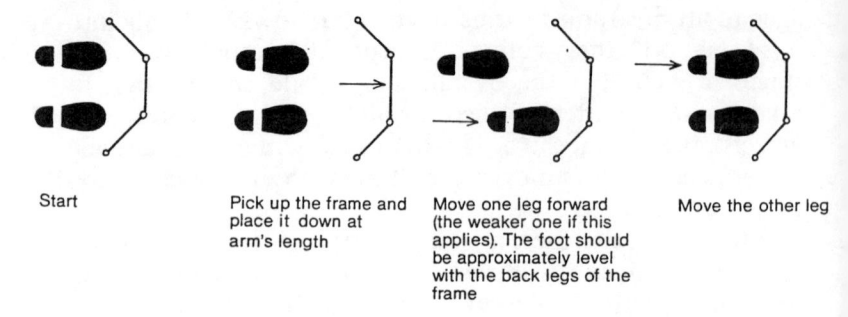

Fig. 8.1 *Gait pattern when using a walking frame*

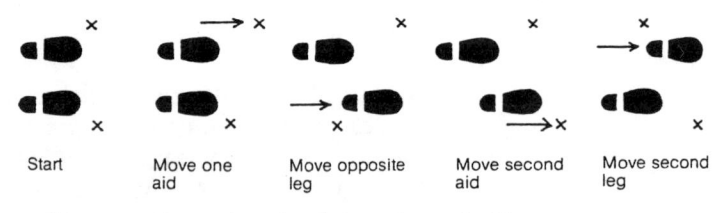

Start | Pick up the frame and place it down at arm's length | Move one leg forward (the weaker one if this applies). The foot should be approximately level with the back legs of the frame | Move the other leg

Fig. 8.2 *Example of a four-point gait. X may represent an axillary or elbow crutch in the early stages of recovery, or a stick in the latter stages*

Start | Move one aid | Move opposite leg | Move second aid | Move second leg

3. Frames. Measure these in the same way as for walking sticks.

Climbing skills

1. Climbing up a single step using an aid
2. Climbing up and down stairs using an aid.

When climbing up a single step such as a kerb, patients are taught to lead with the foot through which they can take most weight and to transfer their weight from the crutches to the foot. The sticks or crutches should then be brought up to be level with the feet.

Most people who are generally fit and in the younger age group feel safer descending stairs on their bottoms. Alternatively, patients can be taught to use handrails or bannisters with one hand and to hold both crutches in the other hand,

THE IMMOBILE INDIVIDUAL IN THE COMMUNITY

using only one of them to take weight. The weight should be taken through the crutch and, with the hand on the handrail, the patient leads with the weaker leg, the stronger leg catching up (see Fig. 8.3). When ascending a flight of stairs, the patient

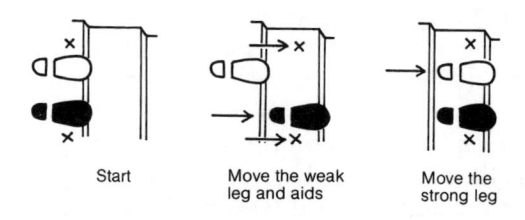

Start   Move the weak leg and aids   Move the strong leg

Fig. 8.3 *Descending stairs using crutches. The shaded area represents either the weak or non weight-bearing leg*

should be instructed to hold one crutch horizontal and to use the other crutch and the handrail; this time, the lead should be taken by the 'good leg' (see Fig. 8.4).

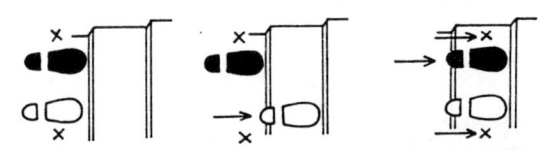

Fig. 8.4 *Ascending stairs using crutches. The shaded area represents either the weak leg or non weight-bearing leg*

Transferring skills

1. Transferring from bed to chair, and the reverse
2. Transferring from chair to toilet, and reverse.

There are various principles that the patient should be taught about transferring from one type of seat to another, whether it be a toilet or a chair. Probably the most important is that the surfaces should be as nearly level and close together as possible. If a gap is unavoidable, it may be bridged by a board. It is also important that the wheels on a wheelchair or commode are firmly locked to prevent any movement. Sometimes, the transfer will be facilitated by the removal of side arms or foot rests.

Whatever techniques are employed by patients to transfer themselves, they are unique to them. However, there are several recognized transfers which may be of help. The corner transfer can be used to move from chair to chair or to a bed. The main principle is that the chair from which the patient is moving should be angled at the chair (bed or toilet) to which the patient is going. At one point, the patient has a hand on both chairs and then sits on the second chair; the final body position is then adjusted. The side transfer may be used with or without a transfer board (see Fig. 8.5). In either case if a wheelchair is used the arm may be removed for ease. Some wheelchairs have a zipped back which can be undone to allow the patient to transfer backwards onto the toilet. This often makes transfer easier in a small toilet where there is not room to position a wheelchair beside the toilet. If the aim is to be independent at transferring on and off the toilet, it should be ensured that the patient is able to reach the toilet paper and the flush.

Daily activities

1. Dressing skills and aids
2. Cooking skills and aids
3. Eating skills and aids.

The availability of aids which may help to restore a patient's ability to be self caring depends on many factors, not least the assessment which the occupational therapist makes of the patient. It may also, unfortunately, depend on the patient's independent financial means, since there are many more than the basic facilities provided available to those who can afford them.

The skills required for the patient to dress and undress independently depend, of course, on the individual, but basic points include ensuring that the patient has adequate room in which to dress, that there is a shelf or chair nearby to put extra clothes on, that all clothes fastenings are in a convenient place (e.g. front fastening bras), and that the clothes are suitable. For example, for female patients who spend all day in a

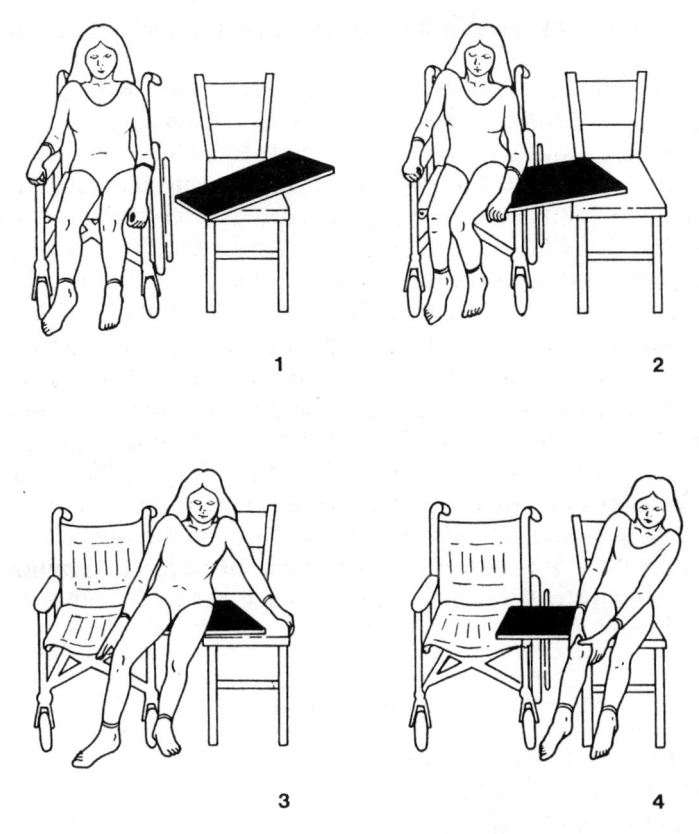

Fig. 8.5 *Using a transfer board. This simple aid may be used in transferring to a toilet or a bed as well as from chair to chair*

wheelchair flared skirts or trousers would be better than tight, straight skirts which ride up and become uncomfortable.

The patient's ability to cook adequately should be assessed by the occupational therapist. Some hospitals have a rehabilitation unit with a well-equipped kitchen which enables patients to try to cook for themselves. It will highlight specific areas in which the patient cannot manage – possibly something very simple such as using a tin opener, peeling potatoes or bending down to open the oven door. The aids available include kitchen utensils with enlarged handles, a tip board to help pour boiling water from the kettle, and adapted plugs to enable those with poor grip to pull an electric plug out of the socket.

To help patients to feed themselves there is a wide range of cutlery with enlarged handles, or there are handles which can be added to everyday cutlery. Cups are available in many shapes to help the disabled, but it is important that the line is drawn on cups which closely resemble children's mugs. Many people find that pottery mugs are too heavy, in which case materials such as melamine are of benefit. There are plates available with a side-guard to enable an individual who has the use of only one arm to push food against it and thus onto a spoon or fork. The advantage of this is that the plate may be of the same design as the ones used by everyone else. There are side-guards available which fit onto plates. These are versatile as they fit many different sizes of plate, but they can look rather degrading.

An outline of the skills and aids that will be required at home should be discussed with the patient and, if appropriate, with the family. However, great care should be taken to ensure that patients do not feel that decisions over their future are being made by other people. Some clinical areas have weekly meetings where occupational therapists and physiotherapists meet with the medical social worker, doctors and nurses to discuss impending discharges. These meetings are particularly helpful when there are some problems over the discharge of a patient which need to be discussed. The major disadvantage is that the patient is not present to hear what is said about them, but possibly this is an area for progress in the future, especially if the self care philosophy is fully adopted.

Before the patient is discharged, it should be arranged for the patient, accompanied by the occupational therapist, to visit the home to see what adaptations will be required. If, during the early stages of the patient's rehabilitation, it becomes obvious that major work will be required, the occupational therapist may need to make a visit alone or with a colleague so that action can be taken well in advance.

In the case of a patient being discharged home while still requiring specific nursing care, the contact between the community and ward staff is crucial to ensure continuity of care. In recognition of this, many clinical areas invite community staff into the ward meetings so that they can familiarize themselves with the needs of the patient and meet the patient before discharge. In some spinal units, community staff actually visit the unit and care for the patient before discharge. Patients who have suffered a spinal injury that has left them hemiplegic or paraplegic will have built up such a rapport with the unit staff over the 9–12 months as in-patients that they inevitably will feel very vulnerable after discharge. By having community staff in the ward area, both the patient's fears and the community nurse's apprehensions may be reduced. This will benefit the patient in the long run. The aim of all these systems is that there should not be a cut-off point where a patient might slip through the net between hospital and home and not receive the care they require. For this to be effective, the relationship between hospital and community staff must be one of give and take and of professionals working for the benefit of the patients. In the past, community staff have sometimes been regarded by hospital-based staff as the 'Cinderella' service. However, steady progress is now being made in improving working relationships between hospital and community staff, although much remains to be achieved. If both groups were to work with the same philosophy or model of nursing, for example the self care model of Orem, continuity of care would benefit enormously.

FACILITIES AVAILABLE IN THE COMMUNITY FOR THOSE WITH A MOBILITY PROBLEM

In 1983, Gormley and Walters completed a research project on the mobility needs of the disabled in the community. This project examined various aspects of the life of an individual with a mobility problem. The conclusions reached showed that the disabled venture out infrequently and that when they do it is usually to friends or for essential shopping. Another finding was the rather haphazard way in which provision for the disabled had developed, with the result that even professionals were not entirely sure where to go for specific help. Gormley suggested that an organization similar to the Consumers Association should be set up to monitor aids for the disabled. The income of the disabled was found to be much lower than the national average, and the financial help available did not redress the balance in most cases. The final finding of the project was that very few of the disabled had any idea of their legislative rights under the *Chronically Sick and Disabled Person's Act*, 1970.

Figure 8.6 shows many of the facilities that are available for those with a mobility problem in the community. It emphasizes the large number of different agencies with which the disabled individual may have to deal in order to ensure that all their needs are met. This difficult situation has been made worse by the historical assumption that those with a physical disability (which includes a mobility problem) will depend on charitable aid for much of their support in the community (Blaxter, 1987). Another problem highlighted by Blaxter was that provision of the most expensive goods available for the disabled, such as adapted cars, was in the hands of high-status medical professionals who prescribed them according to the patient's perceived needs. This would be an effective way of reducing the number of requests for such facilities. For many, the bureaucratic system seems too much to handle.

A further difficulty that may be encountered by those with a mobility problem is the geographical position of the various offices which have to be visited. For an individual whose condition has deteriorated at home and who now requires, for example, alterations to the toilet, the agencies involved may be:

1. The general practitioner
2. The community occupational therapist
3. An official from the social security office
4. The housing department (administrative)
5. The housing department (builders)
6. A social worker
7. A community nursing sister
8. The environmental health officer.

However, having painted this rather bleak picture of the difficulties in obtaining help in the community, there are facilities available and an important nursing function is to

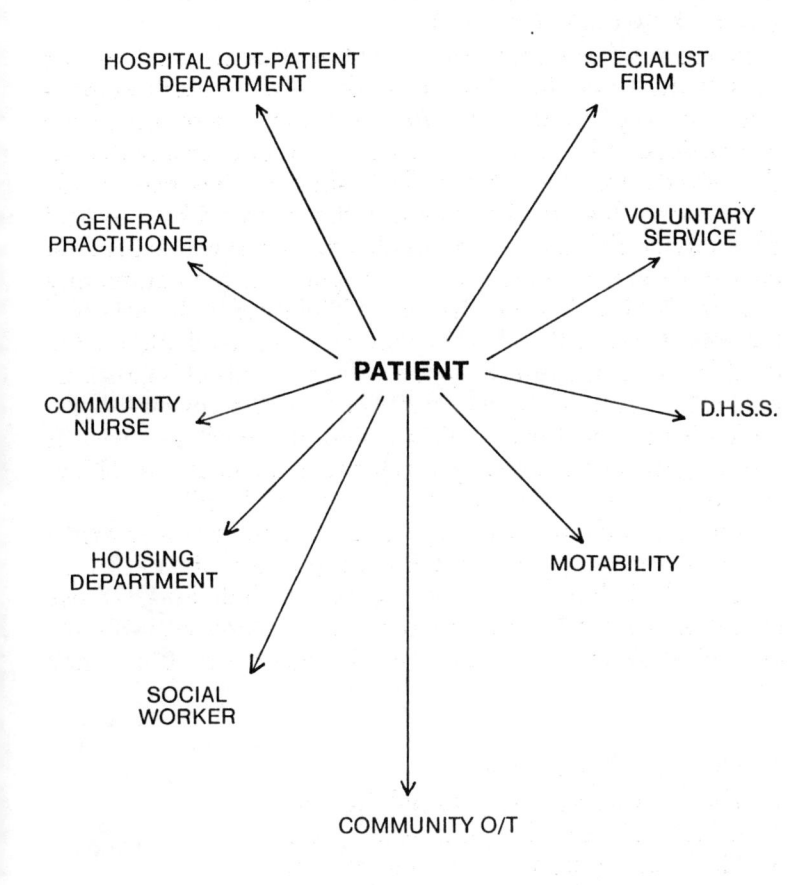

Fig. 8.6 *Some of the many agencies a patient with a mobility problem in the community may need to contact to receive the benefits available*

help patients to use the system so that they can improve the quality of their lives. Some of the more well-used facilities are:

1. *The community physiotherapist*, who is usually based at a hospital but works for a specific general practitioner. In an article describing the role of the community physiotherapist, Lamont and Langford (1980) suggest two reasons why patients may be referred to them, one is because the patient is too sick to travel to a hospital and the other because the family requires help and advice about how to care for the patient. This advice may also be for the patient of course and may be the continuation of the care given in hospital, such as ensuring that the patient uses the walking aids safely or continues to transfer in such a way that there is no risk of skin shearing over the buttocks and pressure sores developing.
2. *The community occupational therapist*, who may work in many guises. The rehabilitation officer may be an occupational therapist as may the disabled living adviser and occupations officer. Jay (1985) suggests that this usually occurs when the occupational therapist is employed by the social services and is able to enjoy a slightly higher salary than that of the NHS counterparts. The major part of all occupational therapists' work now involves helping disabled individuals with their activities of daily living. The Disabled Living Foundation is staffed mainly by occupational therapists and, together with the Aids Centres and travelling exhibition, provides somewhere for the disabled to go to try out various aids and get advice on the spot. The National Aids for the Disabled Exhibition (NAIDEX), at which manufacturers display their goods, occurs twice a year and again gives both the disabled and those caring for them an opportunity to see what has become available. The number of occupational therapists working in the community has increased dramatically since the passing of the *Chronically Sick and Disabled Person's Act* in 1970, yet it is still often seen as a crisis role and many occupational therapists feel they would like to have greater follow-up care of patients whom they have helped. For those with a mobility problem and who are unable to return to work, day centres can help in developing an interest in leisure

activities to try to reduce the level of boredom and frustration. They also provide the individual with a place to meet others with similar problems. Unfortunately such facilities as these are under severe financial pressure in the current climate.
3. *The community nursing service* which will be involved with any specific nursing care a patient may require on discharge, and will also coordinate the medical care being provided by the general practitioner. The community nurse will have to work as much with the family and significant others as with the patient since a great deal of her input will be in Orem's educational/supportive role.
4. *Community chiropodists* who are an underrated commodity. They are few in number and yet meet a tremendous need. For those who have a mobility problem which leads to parasthesia and reduced circulation to the feet, foot care must be of the highest order, while for others their disability may prevent them from carrying out routine footcare themselves. If sores and toe-nail deformities are to be avoided, so that orthoses or footwear can still be worn, professional help is required. Many people with a mobility problem place their feet unevenly on the ground and so are likely to develop corns and callouses which make mobilizing even more painful and difficult. The patient in the community may be referred to the chiropodist via the community nurse or general practitioner, but will have to be warned that there could be a long wait.
5. *Social workers*, are often regarded as the linchpin of services in the community which are not directly medical, although of course they often work in close liaison with general practitioners and health visitors. Very often, social workers can also be seen to be the patient's (client's) advocate and to fight on his or her behalf to ensure all that to which the disabled individual is entitled.

A simple example of how a social worker can help concerns obtaining disabled stickers for the car to allow the disabled person access and parking rights. This can make a tremendous difference to the accessibility of shops and shopping for those with a mobility problem. The social worker should also be able to provide a list of voluntary organizations that may be able to help either

financially or in a practical way by providing a holiday placement in a specifically designed holiday flat or home.
6. *The Department of Health and Social Security* (DHSS), which deals with many of the financial enquiries an individual with a mobility problem may have, but which also sets guidelines for provisions that should be made by the health authority for the disabled in the community. It is important that nurses and social workers ensure that the patient obtains the maximum entitlement from Social Security.
7. *Charitable organizations* in many cities and towns, which are run specifically to make people aware of their legal and financial rights within the welfare state. The social work department will have the local addresses.

This is not an exhaustive list by any means as there are many facilities available in local communities which are relevant only to those localities. However, it does highlight the number of different agencies that may be involved in the care of an individual in the community, and therefore the possibility that the patient may fall between some of these agencies, much to their detriment. Nursing staff in hospitals should be making the patient and family aware of the different agencies that can help them after discharge in much the same way the community nurses do.

FINANCIAL ASSISTANCE FOR THE DISABLED

The financial aid that is available for the disabled in the community falls into several discrete categories. The DHSS sets guidelines on what is available, but it is left to the local authority to decide exactly who gets what. Once again, the allowances come from many different sources locally, so that the individual with a mobility problem will need to look carefully at the help being received and that entitled. This may come as a great shock for someone who has never had to rely on 'government handouts' in the past and who feels it is a request for charity rather than a civil right. While in hospital, patients are cushioned from the harsh realities of the outside

THE IMMOBILE INDIVIDUAL IN THE COMMUNITY

world, but once discharged it can be more of a struggle for the patient to get what is rightfully deserved.

Mobility allowance

This is intended for people who are unable or almost unable to walk. It is a weekly cash benefit to help with extra transport costs, such as taxis, to help improve the quality of life for those whose mobility is restricted. It is available for individuals aged over five (and so it could be used to help take a child on holiday or for a day out) and under 65 years, although once a person is receiving the allowance payment, it will be continued until the age of 75 years. The individual must have had the mobility problem for at least six months to be eligible. It is paid at the same flat rate for everyone.

The person applying for the mobility allowance is examined by an independent doctor who assesses the individual's ability to walk with any aid that is usually used. The doctor will look at the distances the individual can walk, as well as the effect the exercise has on the individual, for example breathlessness. This is one of the benefits that is available from the DHSS.

Motability

Motability is a charitable organization that was founded as the result of a Government directive to help those in receipt of a mobility allowance to lease or buy a car. The DHSS has to be authorized to direct the mobility allowance straight to Motability by the individual. Motability run parallel systems. One of these involves leasing the car over four years and paying an advanced rental and special insurance. An annual charge is made by Motability for mileage in excess of 10 000 miles per year. Adaptions for specific disabilities can be made to the car, although these are done at the person's own expense. The alternative system allows the patient to take advantage of a hire-purchase scheme to buy a car, but they must arrange fully comprehensive insurance. Motability may help the disabled person with the deposits for either scheme and in the payment for the adaptations, although these are discretionary and means-tested.

The 'orange badge scheme' is used by all local authorities to help the disabled with their parking problems. The badges are of two types – one to be used when a disabled person is being transported in the car and the other for use when the disabled person drives the car. The penalty for abusing the system is a fine of about £200.

All beneficiaries of the mobility allowance are entitled to vehicle excise duty exemption (VED). Individuals who are too old for mobility allowance may also be entitled to VED under certain circumstances.

Invalidity benefit

This replaces sickness benefit after 28 weeks of sickness. The invalidity pension is paid to those of pensionable age and an invalidity allowance to those who are younger (i.e. up to the age of 60 years for men and 55 years for women).

Supplementary benefit

This is paid to all those who are not in full-time employment and whose income from the various other allowances and benefits does not reach a set minimum. Some benefits, such as mobility allowance and attendance allowance, are no longer counted as income and therefore do not affect the level of supplementary benefit.

Disabled benefit

This benefit is for those who have had an accident at work or who are now unable to work because of a recognized industrial disease. Any employee is entitled to this benefit, which may be paid as a lump sum or a weekly benefit 15 weeks after the accident or after becoming disabled by the disease. The individual must have suffered loss of physical or mental faculty to be entitled to this benefit, which includes gross deformity even though there is no physical impairment. The assessment looks only at the physical and mental faculties and does not take into account the likelihood of a return to work or what the earnings are likely to be. The assessment fixes a level at which the benefit should be paid – if the disablement is assessed at less than 20%, the benefit will

THE IMMOBILE INDIVIDUAL IN THE COMMUNITY

usually be paid as a lump sum, whereas if it is more than 20%, it will be paid as a weekly pension.

Special hardship allowance

This is a special benefit paid to those who, because of their injury or illness, have an assessed disability of less than 100% but are unable to earn a wage comparable with their previous one. The claimant must have been disabled for at least 90 days (15 weeks) and be likely to remain in that state of incapacitation.

Hospital treatment allowance

Individuals receiving a reduced disablement allowance may have it brought up to the full amount while they are receiving in-patient hospital care. Like the disablement allowance, it is available only if the incapacity is due to an industrial accident or disease.

Constant attention allowance

This is available for those who, as the result of an industrial accident or disease, are in need of constant attention.

Exceptionally severe disablement allowance

Those already receiving the above may qualify for this benefit if the need for such attendance is likely to be permanent.

Attendance allowance

This benefit is available for those not receiving constant attendance allowance but who require a high level of help because of a mental or physical handicap. It is paid at two rates – a day allowance and a night allowance. The claimant must have required such help for at least three months to be eligible for the allowance, which is paid at the post office weekly or by direct credit transfer to a bank account.

Invalid care allowance

This is a weekly cash benefit paid to those who care for a minimum of 35 hours a week for an individual who is in receipt of an attendance allowance. To claim this benefit, the carer must not work in paid employment for more than twelve hours per week. It can be paid only to those over 15 years of age and under 65 years for men, or 60 years for women.

Employment provision for those with a mobility problem

The Manpower Services Commission (MSC) which funds the local job centres also provides specialist care for the disabled in the form of the disablement resettlement officer (DRG). These individuals may be found at some job centres, although not all. Their specific role is to try to place the disabled into suitable employment. This may be in open employment – all employers have an obligation to employ 3% of their total workforce from those on the disabled register. A recent innovation is that of sheltered placements, in which the MSC will help an employer to employ a disabled individual by sharing the cost. In this way, the employer is seen as a sponsor rather than an employer. In most large cities, there are sheltered workshops which specifically employ a high percentage from the disabled register (66%). Remploy are probably the largest government aided agency, although each factory is supposed to be autonomous. These factories manufacture a wide range of goods but specialize in surgical appliances (bespoke shoes and corsets) and aids for the disabled such as walking frames and commodes.

For those who are recently disabled, the Employment Resettlement Centre will assess individuals to discover their suitability for various types of employment. There are usually skill centres on the same site where new training can occur.

Housing assistance

For those living in council accommodation, there are a few extra financial benefits such as rent and rate allowances, and the housing department will pay for structural alterations. For those in private accommodation, a rate rebate may be available, and any structural alterations that are needed should be paid for by the DHSS. The extent of the alterations that are needed should not be underestimated, for example doors may need widening and steps replacing with ramps.

SUMMARY

There is a broad consensus that in the long term most patients are better off in the community than in hospital, and this clearly applies to patients with mobility problems. We have seen that support falls into two main areas – the health problems that the patient faces and the social problems. It would be a mistake, though, to compartmentalize in this way because a health problem has social consequences and social difficulties will lead to health problems.

In addition to receiving the maximum support from the community and hospital-based nursing services, the patient also needs the physical resources to practise self care. The social worker is the key person here, but there should be close liaison with the community nurse for, as we have said, social and health problems are closely interwoven.

It is to be hoped that in future years governments will make sufficient resources available for community care to realize its full potential for the patient. The government record of the 1980s, however, suggests that community care is seen more as a cheap option and consequently is inadequately resourced. Winston Churchill was once quoted as saying 'Give us the tools and we'll do the job'; the same comment applies to community care today.

References

Blaxter M. (1987). *The Meaning of Disability*. Aldershot: Gower Publishing.
Jay P. (1985). *Help Yourself*. London: Ian Henry Publications.
Lamont P., Langford R. (1980). Community physiotherapy in a rural area. *Physiotherapy*, **66** (1), 8–10.

Bibliography

Chartered Society of Physiotherapists (1975). *Handling the Handicapped*. Published by Woodhead–Faulkner, Cambridge, in association with the Chartered Society of Physiotherapists.

Davies B.D. (1982). *The Disabled Child and Adult*. London: Balliere Tindall.

Davies B.M. (1979). *Community Health Preventative Medicine and Social Services*, 4th edn. London: Balliere Tindall.

Gormley R., Walters L. (1983). *Mobility needs of Disabled People in the UK: A formal sample survey. Handicap in a social world*, ed. Brechin A., Liddiard P., Swain J. Kent, England: Hodder and Stoughton in Association with the Open University Press, 119–127.

McCarthy G., ed. (1984). *The Physically Handicapped Child*. London: Faber and Faber.

Stopford V. (1987). *Understanding Disability*. London: Arnold.

Turner A., ed. (1981). *The Practice of Occupational Therapy*. Edinburgh: Churchill Livingstone.

Index

Acetylcholine 3
Ack M. 134
Action potential 16
Activity programme 93
Act of Parliament: Chronically Sick and Disabled Person's 1970 174, 176
Acute anterior cervical spinal cord syndrome 112
Acute anterior poliomyelitis (infantile paralysis) *see under* poliomyelitis
Aids Centres 176
Aids/skills, self care 170–3 *see also* Appliance departments
  cooking 171–2
  dressing 170–1
  drinking 80, 172
  eating 83, 130, 172
Alternating pressure mattress 51
Ambulant, definition 1
Amelia 156–7
Amputation:
  peripheral vascular disease-induced 121
  traumatic 117–23
Anal sphincter, flaccid 85, 86
Anderson E. 159

Anuria 79
Aperient 139
Appliance departments 81 *see also* Aids/skills, selfcare
Arthrodesis 128
  wedge 156
Ataxic 126, 130
Atelectasis 77
Atherosclerosis 129
Atonic 85
Attendance allowance 181
Auto-immune disease 18
Autonomic nerve fibre 111
Axilla 167

Baird S. 101
Baker C. 147
Basal ganglia 3
Beds/mattresses, permanent mobility problems 89–91
Ben-Schlomo L. 93
Benefits 178–82
Bespoke shoes 182
Bladder control loss 84
  spinal cord injury-induced 112, 116
Bladder training programme 85, 87, 116–17
Blaxter M. 174

INDEX

Bobath B. 124
Bobath method 153
Body image, changes in 100
Bones as levers 5, 6 (fig)
Boredom, immobility-induced 27
Bowel control loss 84
  spinal cord injury-induced 112
Bowel function 85
Brachial plexus 167
Brain:
  blood supply 12 (fig)
  motor area 9
  tumors 15
Braun's frame 58, 59 (fig)
Breathing exercises 77–8
Breathless 78
Broad arm sling 137
Brown-Séquard Syndrome 112
Burke D. 115–16
Bursae 3

C4 116
C7 116
Calcaneum 125
Calcaneum/cuboid 156
Caliper 63, 64 (fig), 113–14, 153
Cannula 149
Cannulating 149
Catheterization:
  long-term 85
  residual 86
  self-performed 86
  short-term 85
  spinal shock during 116
Cauda equina 111, 112
Central sulcus 124
Centrally 76
Cerebellar incoordination 126
  weighted aids 126
Cerebellum 3
Cerebral embolism 12
Cerebral haematoma 12, 13, 15 (fig)
  evacuation 14
Cerebral haemorrhage 11, 12, 128
Cerebral hypoxia 76, 78
Cerebral oedema 13, 123
Cerebral palsy 152–3
  asymmetrical (hemiplegia) 152
Cerebral thrombosis 11
Cerebrospinal fluid sac 154
Cerebrovascular accident (CVA) 10–15, 128–30
Cerebrum, function areas 10 (fig)
Cervical spinal cord syndrome, acute anterior 112
Cervical spine, fracture dislocation 74
Charitable organizations 178
Chemonucleolysis 66
Cheshire Homes 75
Child mobility problems:
  care 133–61
    communication on same level 137–8, 149, 150, 151
    education 135
    parental involvement 135–6
    play needs 134–5
    pre-admission visit 151
    pre-adolescent development stages 133–4
Child mobility problems, permanent 151–60
  congenital handicap:
    emotional development of child 158–60
    mechanical maldevelopment-induced 155–7
    neural maldevelopment-induced 152–5

INDEX *187*

Child mobility problems, temporary 136–51
  fear/anxiety-induced 150–1
  plaster of Paris splint 136–40
  surgery, following 146–50
  traction 140–45
Chiropodist, community *see* community chiropodist
Cholinesterase 3–4
Chronically Sick and Disabled Person's Act 1970 174, 176
Churchill Winston 183
Chymopapain 66
Circle of Willis 11, 12 (fig)
Clarke L. 159
Club foot *see* congenital talipes equinovarus
Colleges of further education 92
Colles' fracture 45
Commode 79, 169
Comminuted fracture 136
Community, immobile individual living in 163–83
  facilities available 173–8
  financial assistance 178–83
    benefits/allowances 178–82
    employment 182
    housing 182–3
  hospital transfer preparation 163–73 *see also under* Discharge
    climbing skills 168–9
    daily activities 170–3
    transferring skills 169–70
    walking skills 166–8
Community care 173–8, 183
  government funding 183
Community care staff/hospital relationship 172–3
Community chiropodist 177

Community home 75, 163
Community nursing service 173, 177
Community occupational therapist 176–7 *see also* Occupational therapist
Community physiotherapist 176 *see also* Physiotherapist
Compartment syndrome 60
Computer use, immobile individual 92
Conductive education 153
Congenital absence of fibula 157
Congenital handicap 106
  children 151–60
  adolescents 159–60
Congenital talipes equinovarus (club foot) 151, 155–6
Constant attention allowance 181
Constipation 84
  prevention 139
Continuity of care 172–3
Contraception education, handicapped adolescent 160
'Conveen' system 85
Corsets 63 (fig), 65, 182
Corticospinal tracts, loss 154
Counter traction 115, 145
Crêpe bandage 140, 141, 149
Crutches 137, 155, 167, 168
  axilliary 166, 167
  elbow 166
Crutches, stair negotiation 169 (figs)
Crutchfield calipers 113 (fig)
Cyanosis 76, 78
Cystogram 116
Cystometrogram 116

Day leg-bag 85

Deep vein thrombosis 23–4, 52, 53–5
  anticoagulant medication 54–5
  risk factors 53–4
Deformities, joints 39–40
  spinal 39
  valgus 39
Dehydration 79, 80
  paralytic ileus-associated 116
Denham pin 47, 49
Department of Health and Social Security (DHSS) 178
Depression:
  immobility-induced 27, 92
  progressive disease assessment-induced 89
  self questioning-induced 107
Detrusor autonomic supply 116
Detrusor mechanism 117
Dietician, fine-bore tube feeding 82–3
Diplegia 153
Disabled benefit 180–1
Disabled Living Foundation 176
Disabled person in community *see* Community, immobile individual living in
Disablement resettlement officer (DRG) 182
Discharge *see also under* Community, immobile individual living in
  education for 94, 99–100, 104
  preparatory visits home 103–4
Discography 66
Disease, progressive
  motor neuron 89
  multiple sclerosis 89
Distraction, gentle 113
Dizepam 117
'Does he take sugar' syndrome 88
Dorner S. 159, 160
Dorsiflexion 124
  loss 144
Duchenne muscular dystrophy 18
Dynamic 76, 102
Dysmelia 156–7
Dyspraxia 125 *see also* Gait

Electrical suction drain 71
Elevation period 137
Embolism 12
  cerebral 12
  fat 12
  pulmonary 53, 78
Employment Resettlement Centre 182
'Encourage fluids' 81
Environmental health officer 174
Epidural anaesthesia 68
Erb muscular dystrophy 18
Eversion deformities 40
Exceptionally severe disablement allowance 181
Extensor 117
Extrapyramidal tract 3

Faeces, manual evacuation 85
Fat embolism 12
Fear/anxiety, children 150–1
Femoral dysmelia 157
Femur:
  fracture 138
  fractured shaft 45, 140, 142
Fibula 144
  congenital absence of 157
Fine-bore tube feeding 80, 82
Fitzpatrick J. 93

Flaccid anal sphincter 85
Flaccid paralysis 111, 127, 154
Flaccidity 9
  spinal cord injury-induced 112
Flexion deformities 119–20
  fixed 153
  plantar 156
Flexor 117
Fluid balance chart 80, 81
Foot drop 128
Formal operational stage 134
Frustration, physical/emotional, immobility-induced 96
Full arm sling 58, 59 (fig)

Gadgets, self care *see* Aids/ skills, self care
Gait 7 *see also* Dyspraxia
  four-point 167, 168 (fig)
  pattern, using frame 168 (fig)
  three-point 167
Gamgee pad 142
Gas gangrene 118
General practitioner 174
Genu valgus (knock knees) 39
Glasgow Coma Scale 123
Goffman E. 101
Goldberg W. 93
Goniometer 38, 39 (fig)
Gormley R. 173
Greengross W. 160
Grieving 121–2
  Parkes' four-stages 121
Gutter frame 166

Haematoma, chronic subdural 13–14
Haemorrhage 118
Halo brace 115
Handicap, congenital 151–60
  mechanical maldevelopment 155–7

neural maldevelopment 152–5
Handicap, definition 158
Hazards:
  patient education 99–100
  prevention 98–100
Head injury 13–15
'Head nurse' 115
Hemimyelomeningocele 155
Hemiplegia 129–30, 152
Hickey J. 92
High arm sling 137
Hilgard E. 100
Hip, congenital dislocation 19, 138
Hip spica 133, 139, 140
  bilateral 134, 138 (fig)
  unilateral 138, 139, 140
Homans' sign 54
Homunculus 10, 11 (fig)
Hospital/community care staff relationship 172–3
Hospital treatment allowance 181
Housing department 174
Humerus, supracondylar fracture 140, 145
Hydrochloric acid 82
Hydrotherapy 117
Hyperextension injury, lateral 112
Hypertonic 153
Hypotension 79, 111, 129
  postural 114
Hypoxia 77, 116
  cerebral 76, 78

Ideopathic muscle imbalance 156
Iliacus muscle 119
Immobile individual living in community *see under* Community, immobile individual living in
Immobile individual, computer

use 92
Immobility 9–28
　assessment 36–40
　effects on patient's life 37–8
　　sexual 96
　nursing care 30–6
　nursing model 36–7
　patient's ability 37
　self care see Self care
　side effects 21–7
　　contractures 26–7
　　deep vein thrombosis 23–4
　　depression/boredom 27
　　muscle wasting 26
　　pressure sores 23
　　pulmonary congestion 25
　　urinary stasis/infection 26
Incontinence 79, 86–7
Independence 74
　diminished by permanent immobility 88
　promotion through self care 92–3
Infantile paralysis (acute anterior poliomyelitis) see under Poliomyelitis
Inflatable ball 125
Inflatable mattress 125
Institutional care, long-term 74
Intercostal muscle 116
Intra-abdominal muscles 80
Intracranial pressure 128
Intravenous fluids 80, 123
Intravenous infusion(s) 69–70, 116
　child with 148–9
Intravenous pyelogram 116
Intravenous stand 137
Invalid care allowance 182
Invalidity benefit:
　allowance 180
　pension 180
Inversion deformities 40

Ischial tuberosity 63, 142, 157

Jay P. 176
Joints:
　anatomy 2–3
　contractures 26–7
　　reduction 124
　deformity
　　arthrodesis 128, 156
　movements 38
　　normal range 38–9
　passive exercises 91–2
　pathological changes 18–21
　stiffness 55–6

Karn M. 133, 134
Kelly 121–2
Kirschner wire 47, 48 (fig)
Knock knees (genu valgus) 39
Kyphosis 39

L1 111
Lamont P. 176
Landouzy Déjérine muscular dystrophy 18
Langford R. 176
Lateral hyperextention injury 112
'Learned helplessness' 88
Leonard B. J. 101
Limb compartments 60
'Lived body' 7
Lordosis 39
Lower motor neurone 3, 4 (fig), 17
　injury 111, 116, 117
Lumbar radiculum 66

McCallum A. T. 135–6
McGill Pain Questionnaire 41, 42
Mackie J. 147
Manksch H. 122

INDEX

Manpower Services Commission (MSC) 182
Manual Evacuation 85
'Marking' on skin 91, 143 *see also* Pressure sores
Mather L. 147
Meninges 154
Meningocele 154
Metal introducer 82
Micturation 84–5
Mobility 1–8
  definition 1
Mobility allowance 179
Mobility goals, patient 93
Mobility skills 167–73
  climbing 168–9
  daily activities 170–3
  transferring 169–70
  walking 166–8
'Mongol' used as abuse 160
Motability 179–80
Motor cortex 124
  function 124–5
Motor neurone disease 89
Motor system 16–17
  pathway interruption 17
Movement 5–7
Movement therapy programme 93
'Multidisciplinary approach' 88–9, 169
Multiple Sclerosis Society 81
Multiple sclerosis 17
Murray D. 115–16
Murray R. L. 101
Muscle:
  shortening, prevention 91
  wasting 26, 111
Muscle imbalance 156
Muscle pump 24
Muscle(s), striped 5
Muscular dystrophy 18
Myasthenia gravis 17, 18
Myelography 65–6

Myelomeningocele 154

Nasogastric tube 83, 116
National Aids for the Disabled Exhibition (NAIDEX) 176
National Association of the Welfare of Children in Hospital (NAWCH) 150
Nerve fibre, myelinated (medullated) 16–17
Nerve root 112
Neural maldevelopment 152–5
Neurogenic bladder 116
Neurological disorders 16–18
Neuromuscular condition 80
Neuromuscular physiology 3–5
Nodes of Ranvier 17
Normalcy, definition 100–1, 104
Nurse-centred/patient-centred care 164
Nursing care, self care emphasis 164
Nursing diagnosis 30
Nutrition, factors preventing self care 82

Occupational therapist 130, 170, 171, *see also* Community occupational therapist
Occupational therapy departments 81
Oedema 105–6, 119
  ankle 105–6
  cerebral 13, 123
  hand 106
  generalized 106
Oliguria 79
Operational stage 134
'Orange badge scheme'

179–80
Orem's self care model 34–6, 75, 163
Orthopaedic traction table, pressure sores induced by 53
Orthosis 128 (fig), 155
Orthotic bracing 61–4
  lower limb 62–3
  upper limb 63
Osmolality 83
Osteoarthritis 3, 19, 20 (fig), 105
Overdistension 85
Oxygen 51

Paediatric glycerine suppository 139
Pain 40–3
  duration 42
  factors affecting assessment 42
  location 41
  postoperative 69
    phantom limb 122–3
  rating scales 41–2
    children 147
  severity 41–2
  stereotypical responses 146–7
  type 40–1
Pain, ache, hurt questionnaire 41
Pain, child in 146–8
Paralytic ileus 115–16
Paraplegia 105
Parasthenia 177
Parkes C. M. 122
Parkinson's disease 3
Passive exercises 91–2, 94
Patella 142
Patient-centred/nurse-centred care 164
Pathological changes 9
Pedal pulse 141

Pelvic band 155
Perineal nerve supply 116
Peripheral vascular disease 121
Periphery (finger/toe nail beds) 76
Permanent immobility:
  congenital handicap, child 151–60
  gradual onset 74–107
  sudden onset 109–31
    patient categories 109–10
Peroneal nerve 144
Perthes' disease 19
Peto Dr Andras 153
PHAB (physically handicapped and able-bodied) 160
Phantom limb 122–3
Physiotherapist 166 *see also* Community physiotherapist
Piaget J. 133, 134, 137
Plantar flexion 129, 156
Plaster care 137–8
Plaster sore 61
Plaster splints 57–61
  plaster of Paris 136–40
Platt report (1959) 135
Play leader 135
Play needs 134–5
Pneumonia 77
Poliomyelitis 17
  acute anterior (infantile paralysis) 127–8
  immunization 127
  spinal paralytic 127
Postural adjustment 125
Pre-operational stage 133–4
Pressure sores 23, 50–3
  incontinence-associated 51–2
  mattress/mattress cover-induced 91
  orthopaedic traction table-induced 53

spinal cord injury-associated 115
splint-induced 139
traction-associated 140, 142–4
Profiling bed 90, 114
Proprioception 112
  loss of 130
Prosthesis:
  above-knee 118
  below-knee 118
  extension 157
  hip supporting 157
  myo-electric 157
Protamine 55
Psoas muscle 119
Psycho-sexual counselling 96
Pulmonary congestion 25
Pulmonary embolism 53, 78
'Push fluids' 81
Pyrexia 79

Quadriplegia 110
Quadriplegic 115, 116
QUEST notion 115, 116

Ragiel C. 133, 134
Redivac drain 70
Reflex:
  spinal 111, 129
  spinal arc emptying 116
  stretch 116
Regional Spinal Cord Injuries Unit 110
Rehabilitation 163, 165
  units 165, 171
  see also Community, immobile individual living in
Remploy factories 182
Renal calculi 26
Residual catheterization 86
Respiration 75–8
Respirator, mechanical 76
Resuscitation ABC 123

Rheumatoid arthritis 3, 19–21, 22 (fig), 107
  affect on domestic routine 79
  fluid intake 80
Rollator 153, 155, 167
Roper's model of nursing 33–4
Roy's adaptation model 31–3

Sabin vaccine 127
Scoliosis 39
Self care aids/skills *see* Aids/skills, self care
Self care requisites
  developmental 104–5
  health deviation 105–7
    behaviour 106–7
    body structure 105–6
    function 106
  universal 75–104
    activity/rest balance 88–95
    air intake 75–8
    excrement control 84–8
    fluid intake 79–81
    food intake 81–4
    hazard prevention 98–100
    normalcy promotion 100–3
    social activity/solitude balance 95–8
Self-catheterization 86
Self-image 100
Self medication 99, 100
Self questioning 106–7
Sensorimotor stage 133
Sensory loss 79, 155
Serial plaster cylinders 124
Severe head injury 123–6
Sexual counselling, congenitally handicapped individual 160 *see also* Psycho-sexual counselling

Shakespeare R. 101–2, 103
Sheepskin pads/bootees 51
Short M. 93
'Significant others' 76, 86, 94
Sjögren syndrome 19
Skin extension 46, 140, 142
'Sleek' 139
Social worker 177–8
Spastic paralysis 152
'Spastic' used as abuse 160
Spasticity 9, 111
   patterns 117
Special hardship allowance 181
Spica *see* hip spica
Spina bifida 153–5, 159
   occulta 154
Spinal anaesthesia 67–8
Spinal arc emptying reflex 116
Spinal brace 89
Spinal cord injury (lesion) 17, 86, 110–17
   complete transection 111–12
   incomplete lesion 112
      syndromes 112
Spinal cord injury (lesion)
   prevention of associated complications 115–17
   vertebral column alignment 112–15
      turning method 114–15
Spinal investigation 64–6
Spinal ligaments 110, 111 (fig)
Spinal paralytic poliomyelitis 127
Spinal reflex 111, 129
Spinal shock 113
Spinal unit 117, 173
Splint/splinting 89, 127, 129, 136–40
'Spoon-fed' 83
Sputum 77–8
Steinmann's pin 47
Sternum 115

Steroids 107
Stigma 101
Stoke Egerton bed (electric turning) 89, 113
Stopford V. 158
Stretch reflex 116, 117
Stroke 75, 129
Stryker turning frame 90–1, 113
Stump bandaging 119
Subcutaneous elasticity loss 79
Supplementary benefit 180
Support groups:
   cerebrovascular accident 130
   severe head injury 126
Supracondylar fracture 140, 145
Suprapubic catheter 85
Surgery, immobilization following 69–71
Symphysis pubis 115
Synapse 17 (fig)

T12 111
Taggliacozzo D. L. 122
Temporary immobilization 44–71
   child 136–51
Tendons 5
Tentorial herniation 13, 14 (fig)
Tetanus 118
Thalidamide 156
Thomas' splint 48 (fig), 56, 143, 144 (fig)
Thoracic band 155
Thrombus 53
Tibia, comminuted fracture 136
Tilt table 124, 125
Tincture of benzoin 140
Toe-sprung orthosis 128
Tongs 113–14
Total paralysis 74

INDEX

Tracheostomy 76, 77
  long-term silver 77
  short-term plastic 77
Traction 45–53 *see also* Counter traction
  anaesthetic during application 141
  analgesia during 52
  Dunlop 145
  fixed skin 142–4
    removal of 144
  Gallows (Bryant's) 140–2
  halopelvic (halo brace) 115
  halter 49–50
  manual 142
  pelvic 50
  problems 50–7
    deep vein thrombosis 52, 53–5
    inability to use toilet facilities adequately 56–7, 142
    joint stiffness 55–6
    pressure sores 50–3, 141, 142–3
  skeletal 47–9
    skull 113
  skin 46–7
Traction, child in 140–5
Transfer techniques:
  corner 170
  side 170, 171 (figs)
Trauma unit 117
Traumatic amputation 117–23
  phantom limb 122–3
  postoperative care 119–20
  types 118–19
'Trigger point' 117

Ulnar styloid 167
Underseal drain 71

United Nations 158
Upper motor neuron 3, 4 (fig), 17
  injury 111, 116–17
Urinary stasis/infection 26
'Urosheath' 85

Valgus deformities 39
Varus deformities 40
Vasomotor control, loss 111
Vehicle excise duty exemption (VED) 180
Velafix dressings 70, 149
Vertebra fracture 111
Vertebrae, malformation 153
Vertebral column alignment 112–15
  turning methods 114–15
Viscid secretions 77
Visual Analogue Scale 41
Vitamin K 55
Volkmann's ischaemic contracture 62 (fig)

Walking 5–7
  spina bifida sufferer 155
Walking aids 165–8
Walsh M. 123
Walters L. 173
Ward teacher 135
Wedge arthrodesis 156
Which Report (1980) 151
Why me? 106–7
'Will I be able to walk again?' 131
Wong D. 147
World Health Organization (WHO) 158
Wound contamination 118
Wound drains 70–1, 119
  child with 149–50